NURSING INTIMACY

An Ethnographic Approach to
Nurse–Patient Interaction

NURSING INTIMACY

An Ethnographic Approach to Nurse–Patient Interaction

JAN SAVAGE PhD RGN

Lecturer, Institute of Advanced Nursing Education,
Royal College of Nursing

Staffordshire University
School of Health
Royal Shrewsbury Hospital (North)

SCUTARI PRESS
London

A division of Scutari Projects Ltd, the publishing company of the Royal College of Nursing.

First published 1995

British Library Cataloguing in Publication Data

Savage, Jan
Nursing Intimacy: Ethnographic Approach
to Nurse-Patient Interaction
I. Title
610.730699

ISBN 1–873853–26–2

Typeset by Florencetype Ltd, Stoodleigh, Devon
Printed at Redwood Books, Trowbridge, Wiltshire.

Contents

Foreword

Over the last few years, an expanding body of research evidence has begun to highlight the value of nursing care. This evidence confirms what nurses have known for many years – that nursing care helps more patients to get better more quickly. The research also shows that nursing care is value for money.

To the people who receive skilled nursing care, the value of nursing is self-evident. But traditionally nurses themselves have had great difficulty in articulating what is special about what they do – particularly as so often the highest art of nursing is making it look and feel as if people are not being 'nursed' at all.

In this account, Jan Savage identifies the relationship between nurse and patient as a crucial element in the effectiveness of nursing care. The experiences of the nurses described in this account highlight the therapeutic value of nursing where personal 'closeness' to the patient forms an integral part of the overall care. It looks at what nurses themselves mean by close relationships and what they think the relationship will achieve for patients.

The study also looks at the way in which nurses experience relationships with patients. When I was studying psychology, I discovered the work of Isabel Menzies. She recognised the pain and anxiety which is present in every hospital and how difficult it was for nurses, particularly the young and inexperienced. She also described how we used rigid and ritualistic systems of task allocation as a defence against our own involvement and to enable us to manage difficult and emotional situations.

For experienced nurses, the continuous stress of working with people facing pain and death can produce an obsessive need to stick to rules and procedures. As Menzies pointed out, this can make any reorganisation of care particularly hard to swallow.

Jan Savage's study suggests that nurses who are prepared to use closer relationships with patients therapeutically, managing these relationships skilfully through the use of touch, humour and body posture, did not find the relationships as stressful as might be assumed. Indeed, because of the reciprocal nature of close nurse–patient relationships, some nurses found support rather than stress within these relationships.

What was found to be stressful however was inadequate staffing levels, lack of support staff and stability. Where nurses are free to develop their own approach to managing care and where they can practise with greater autonomy, they are able to achieve greater continuity and a higher standard of care with far less stress than would be the case in a more managed, task-orientated environment.

This certainly tallies with some recent research carried out in the magnet hospitals in the United States where nurses who are given greater autonomy to manage patient care are able significantly to reduce mortality rates and improve patient recovery rates. Consequently these hospitals are able to attract more nurses as well as more patients and more money.

Finally Jan Savage considers the nature of 'nursing knowledge' and how it is learned. She points out that there is very little research material available in this area. As new technology and the advent of day care and key hole surgery transform health care in this country, I believe that this 'knowledge' will mean the difference between success and failure wherever people are cared for; the difference between feeling like a person and feeling like a patient.

While nurses have become more successful in getting the message about the value of nursing across in an increasingly cost-conscious health care environment in recent years, finely articulating what makes nursing care so special is perhaps the next step on the road to winning the arguments. *Nursing Intimacy* is a fascinating study and an effective tool for nurses to demonstrate their central role in tomorrow's health service.

CHRISTINE HANCOCK
GENERAL SECRETARY, RCN

Acknowledgements

This book could not have been written without the help and encouragement of a large number of people. Pam Smith has been involved from the earliest moments of the research process and encouraged me to publish; my heartfelt thanks go to her for her emotional and intellectual labour. Thanks are also due to Karen Greenwood, Meg McDonald and Shelagh Sparrow who, in different ways, provided more support than they probably realise.

To Gene Feder, I can offer no greater accolade than to thank him for nursing me along and for his close reading of numerous drafts. Very special thanks are also due to Ben and Josh Feder for comfort and cheer, as well as understanding beyond their years.

To retain the anonymity of the research setting and those who took part in the research, many people I am grateful to will have to remain unnamed; these include nurse managers, staff in the college of nursing and Directorate of Quality Assurance where I was based, the local Nurses' Research Network, ward clerks, pharmacists, occupational therapists and medical and ancillary staff. I hope they are already aware of how much I valued their time and assistance.

Finally, I must thank the nurses on both wards in the study for their help, for their tolerance and for teaching me so much. I should take this opportunity to say that their commitment to patient care and to the development of nursing was inspiring, especially in view of the relentless change and uncertainty they had to deal with. The wards no longer exist as I describe them, and the staff are scattered, but I hope they feel that the following account suggests something of what they achieved and shows how much their endeavour was admired.

JAN SAVAGE

To the nurses of 'Smith' and 'Jones' Wards,
wherever they may be

1

Introduction

This book has arisen from a one-year research project concerned with a form of nursing innovation that is widely referred to as the 'new nursing' (Salvage 1990). One of the main features of this approach to nursing care is the emphasis placed on the therapeutic potential of nurses' personal involvement with patients. This involvement has often been referred to in the 'new nursing' literature as 'closeness'. This study aimed to explore how nurses understand the notion of 'closeness' and to assess the support they might need where 'close' relationships with patients are encouraged.

CLOSENESS AND CONTINUITY OF CARE

My interest in this area had two points of origin. The first was a concern that unrealistic demands might be made of nurses who adopted this approach. My own nurse training took place when task allocation was the norm and emotional involvement with patients was strenuously discouraged, not always by our nurse tutors but certainly by the majority of ward sisters and what were then called assistant matrons. I was intrigued, therefore, when I returned to nursing after a break of some years to find not only the organisation of nursing care, but also the ethos guiding nurses' interaction with patients and clients, greatly changed. In the literature concerning the 'new nursing', a link is assumed between continuity of care and the nature of the nurse–patient relationship; care that is continuously planned and provided, as far as possible, by a single nurse is thought to allow the development of a 'close' relationship, and it is from this 'closeness' between nurse and patient that a therapeutic potential emerges. While the meaning of 'closeness' is rarely made explicit in such literature, it appears to refer implicitly to emotional understanding and commitment, at least on the part of the nurse. As such, the promotion of 'closeness' would seem to run counter to earlier approaches to nursing care in which nurses were encouraged to distance themselves from patients as a form of self-protection (Jourard 1964, Menzies 1970).

1

At the same time, the emphasis on 'closeness' in new nursing initiatives has to be seen in the context of broader changes taking place in the National Health Service (NHS), most notably its restructuring along the lines of a market economy. The introduction of competition within the NHS has exacerbated a long-standing tension in the system between what is wanted, on the one hand, and what is spent, on the other (Swales 1994). According to Swales, this tension was in the past mitigated largely by the goodwill and dedication of NHS staff, working in what was undeniably an inefficient service but one that had nonetheless remained viable. Now 'the commercial model is being pursued relentlessly but without the flexibility or the resources of the commercial world', with the result of increasing stress on staff responsible for clinical care (Swales 1994, p.247).

NURSES' MANAGEMENT OF 'CLOSENESS'

Thus, changes in nursing ideology, together with the restructuring of the context in which nursing occurs, provided the framework for this research. Such changes prompted a concern that a greater *opportunity* for continuity of care would not necessarily be matched by a consideration of what sustained patient contact meant for nurses. This study aimed to discover whether or not nurses received adequate support where they provided continuity of care, and what form of support they required. Parallel to this, it seemed important to consider whether continuity of care went beyond mere rhetoric. For example, did nurses *really* become 'involved' with their patients, as the protaganists of the 'new nursing' have suggested, or was 'closeness' no more a regular and strategic feature of nursing care than it was in the past?

Such concerns seemed to have relevance beyond the 'new nursing'. Irrespective of the philosophy or organisational mode they wish to adopt, continuity of care has become an important objective for all nurses following the introduction of the Patient's Charter and the 'named nurse' initiative. Put another way, attempts to provide continuity of care occur now not only within grass roots initiatives by nurses, but also as a response to 'top down' imperatives from policy-makers and purchasers. Yet, where continuity of care is imposed, rather than actively promoted by nurses, it may well become a meaningless notion, besides increasing the stress that nurses experience. Concerns of this nature provided much of the impetus for this research, while the precise research questions that informed the study and its methodological approach can be found at the end of Chapter 2.

THE POTENTIAL OF ANTHROPOLOGY

The other point of origin for the research lies in my training as an anthropologist and a subsequent desire to show the relevance of anthropology for nursing theory and research. It was not by chance that my attention was drawn to nurses' references to 'closeness'. In a previous study of English perceptions of kinship and procreation, I had found that a notion of 'closeness' that referred to an emotional intimacy was central to understanding family or 'blood' relationships (Savage 1991). Before this, 'closeness' in European and American kinship studies had been largely neglected by anthropologists or was widely assumed to refer to similarity of bodily substance, such as genetic material. I was intrigued to see 'closeness' being used by nurses to refer to an occupational relationship and to see that the meaning of the term was still taken for granted. At the beginning of the study, there was little reason to suspect that there was a connection between the two notions of 'closeness'; one referred to the discrete domain of kinship and the other to the domain of nursing. However, during the research, kinship relations emerged as potential models for nurse–patient relationships and the giving of care. Moreover, it seems that the cultural construct of 'closeness' plays an important part in the structuring of relationships across a number of domains.

In terms of the study's findings, very briefly, these suggest that 'closeness' is understood as a form of rapport which allows self-disclosure or 'openness'. Experienced nurses in the study employed a range of 'strategies', such as the use of touch, humour and, particularly, body posture, to promote and manage their 'closeness' with patients. The self-disclosure that 'closeness' prompted was seen by nurses to form the central component of the therapeutic process that characterised 'the new nursing'. Often, this disclosure of the self was reciprocal: it required the nurse as well as the patient to be 'open'. Yet, at least for nurses, self-disclosure need not occur verbally – it could be effected through the body. Not surprisingly perhaps, the extent to which 'closeness' and self-disclosure were features of the nurse–patient relationship appeared to be associated not so much with the organisational mode used by nurses, but with the support they received. However, this support took many forms; nurses put less emphasis on the importance of counselling and, instead, stressed the necessity of adequate staffing levels and ancillary services, a stable workforce, appropriate training, and recognition and endorsement from managers and medical colleagues.

THE IMPORTANCE OF CONTEXT

The study's findings, therefore, fall into two broad groups, which have particular relevance, if not poignancy, in the face of changes that are currently taking place in the delivery of health care. The first group of findings is concerned with the provision of what at least some nurses perceived as high-quality nursing care and how the ability to offer this care could not be divorced from the overall context (including resources) in which care was provided. In this respect, this monograph can be seen as a historical document, in that nurses' practice on both wards in the study has changed considerably since the study's completion because of the crisis in resourcing that is occurring in the NHS and the public sector overall. One ward in the study, for example, a nursing development unit which based its care on the importance of the nurse–patient relationship, has changed beyond recognition. This ward was initially well resourced in terms of staffing levels, post-registration training opportunities and support from nurse managers. Yet, as I discuss in the final chapter, changes in resources and the pressure to provide a 'cost-effective' service have led to the collapse of innovative practice and a return to a more 'managerial–medical' (Hart 1991) style of practice, which gives less value to specifically nursing skills.

NURSES' NON-VERBAL KNOWLEDGE

The second group of findings help to make visible some of the elements of nursing that generally go unrecognised, the very nursing skills that are downplayed in current NHS reforms which stress efficiency and measurable outcome. The era of the 'new nursing' is one marked by a recognition of the role of non-verbal knowledge in the provision of care, and, increasingly, nurses – particularly expert nurses – claim to base their actions on intuition or experience (Young 1987, Meutzel 1988) or on 'knowing the patient' through the nurse's everyday practices (Lawler 1991, MacLoed 1993). There is, however, little appropriate vocabulary available to nurses to express this aspect of their work. The findings of this study, I believe, help to increase our understanding of nurses' intuition and embodied knowledge through focusing on their non-verbal behaviour and non-literal language (their use of metaphor and irony, for example). In addition, the methods used to study nurses' non-clinical, non-measurable practice may be of interest to other researchers.

The difficulties of researching what it is that nurses 'know' and how they come to know it have been recognised but are only just beginning to be addressed (see for example Lawler 1991, MacGuire 1991, Meerabeau 1992). My focus on 'closeness' meant that I was attempting to study an aspect of nursing that nurses would probably find difficult to articulate. I was, therefore, interested in using a methodological approach that made allowance for this by offering a possible means of access to tacit forms of knowledge.

In order to examine those aspects of nurses' knowledge that are grounded in the mundane events and lived experience of everyday life, I opted for an ethnographic approach, based on participant observation augmented by informal and semi-structured interviews. The theoretical perspective underlying this approach is one propounded by the anthropologist Michael Jackson (1989), that of 'radical empiricism', in which bodily participation and use of all the senses (not merely sight) are made central. As such, it seems a particularly appropriate approach for a study in which the lived body is not only a focus of care (Lawler 1991) but, arguably, a means of effecting care. As nursing knowledge is increasingly recognised to be only partially dependent on language for its development or transmission (Kitson 1987, Young 1987, Benner and Wrubel 1989), a radical empiricist approach may offer a way of gaining access to the non-verbal, embodied knowledge that nurses hold. Moreover, through using this approach, I hope to indicate the relevance of anthropology in increasing our understanding of nursing.

FINALLY ...

There are two final points to make about the study. First, the vast majority of interaction I observed occurred between female nurses and male patients. This reflected sex ratios in general: the large majority of nurses on both wards in the study were female, and patients were predominantly male. When speaking generally of nurses and patients, I therefore refer to nurses as 'she' and patients as 'he', for the sake of simplicity.

Second, some readers may find the term 'new nursing' questionable where it refers to modes of organising care (such as primary nursing) in which continuity is promoted. The work of psychiatric nurses, for example, or nurses working in the community, may have pre-empted aspects of 'new nursing' philosophy and practice. I have often heard such nurses object that, as a proselytising movement, the 'new nursing' has been biased towards hospital-based care. This study, unfortunately, does nothing to address this trend, in that it focuses exclusively on nursing within the hospital context. Moreover, some of the arguments that I shall make, particularly about how nurses transform the nature of space from public to private, are specific to the hospital or institutional context and would be unlikely to apply in the community, given, for example, that nurses enter clients' private space, largely on the client's terms. However, although different contexts may have different implications for the way in which nurse–patient relationships may develop, I hope that the following account of the complexities and significance of nurse–patient interaction will, nonetheless, have some general relevance for all nurses as well as others who have an interest in nursing and health care generally.

2

Changes in Nursing and Nurse–Patient Interaction

Within contemporary nursing in the UK, the relationship between nurse and patient is widely understood to be of central importance to the provision of quality nursing care (Pearson 1988, Ersser and Tutton 1991). However, this has not always been the case. Until recently, the potential of the nurse–patient relationship was highly constrained. Medical diagnosis and treatment provided the cornerstones of nursing knowledge and ideology, and it has been suggested that, within this scheme, the patient was viewed as essentially a biological body to be observed by the nurse (Armstrong 1983). Although the approach within other branches of nursing may have been rather different (see Altschul 1972 for example), general nurses were encouraged to maintain an emotional distance from their patients (Menzies 1970, Hockey 1976). May (1991) has suggested that this stems from the emergence of nursing as a vocation fit for young women from the upper classes and from associated ideas about the ways in which nurse–patient relationships might be desexualised despite the necessity for physical intimacy.

Traditionally, the work of nurses was organised according to task allocation and so that, as seniority increased, a nurse moved away from 'dirty work' or 'basic care' to more technical tasks requiring less intimacy with patients (Lawler 1991). Task allocation also had the perceived advantage of protecting nurses from anxiety, by reducing the contact and involvement they had with patients (Menzies 1970).

The work of Menzies is of particular relevance for this study as it represents a turning point in understanding nurse–patient interaction and its relationship to nursing organisation. Based at a London teaching hospital, Menzies found a high level of tension, distress and anxiety among nurses, indicated, for example, by a high turnover of senior staff, high numbers of students withdrawing from training and a high sickness rate.

One source of nurses' distress was seen as largely unavoidable (Menzies 1970, p.5); nursing, by the very nature of the job, is inherently stressful:

Nurses are in constant contact with people who are physically ill or injured, often seriously. The recovery of patients is not certain and will not always be complete. Nursing patients who have incurable diseases is one of the nurse's most distressing tasks. Nurses are confronted with the threat and the reality of suffering and death as few lay people are. Their work involves carrying out tasks which, by ordinary standards, are distasteful, disgusting, and frightening.

However, Menzies felt that although 'by the nature of her profession the nurse is at considerable risk of being flooded by intense and unmanageable anxiety' (1970, p.9), the nature of nursing did not, by itself, account for the high level of anxiety apparent in nurses. The very techniques used by nurses to contain and modify anxiety appeared to constitute part of the problem. These included 'splitting up the nurse–patient relationship' through task allocation, and 'denial of the significance of the individual', characterised by nurses' references to patients as, for example, 'the liver in bed 10'. There was often an implicit operational policy of 'detachment', evident in the assumption that a nurse would not mind moving from ward to ward, or even from hospital to hospital without notice (Menzies 1970, p.14):

> The pain and distress of moving, of breaking stable and continuing relationships are implicitly denied by the system although often stressed personally by people (including senior nurses who initiate such moves) within the system.

Thus, Menzies suggested that the stress inherent within nursing was compounded by an organisational structure and ethos that persistently worked against the development of a social relationship between nurse and patient.[1]

Later studies of nurse–patient communication continued to show 'distancing' as a feature of at least some nurses' work. For example, Macleod Clark's (1983) review of research in a variety of nursing contexts described a persistent lack of social conversation between nurses and patients; communication largely corresponded with the giving of instrumental care. Conversation tended to be superficial, with nurses channelling conversation away from difficult issues or failing to take the opportunity to talk with patients when they were not busy. Macleod Clark's own study of the content and structure of nurse–patient conversations on male and female surgical wards concluded that (p.53):

> nurse–patient conversations were limited both in quantity and quality. Nurses displayed little evidence of using skills which encourage communication although many examples were identified of nurses using strategies which may block or discourage communication.

Similarly, Smith (1992) provides evidence that, as recently as the mid-1980s, the ward sister who espoused the development of personal relationships between nurses and patients as a central aspect of nursing might be regarded as eccentric. While the nursing process had been introduced in order to allow nurses to care for patients rather than carry out tasks, Smith found that many students would avoid continuity of care because of their repeated exposure to emotionally demanding experiences without the support of more senior nurses. As one first-year student told her (p.132):

> I came into nursing to care for people. I expected to care for them in pain and when they were dying. What I didn't expect was that the system doesn't always let me do it in the way I want to.

Low levels of job satisfaction among nurses, discontent with task-oriented nursing and the superficial relationships between nurses and patients prompted the introduction of the nursing process and the stress on individualised patient care (de la Cuesta 1983). Yet the nursing process did not necessarily, of itself, bring about continuity of care and more meaningful nurse–patient interaction. Thus new initiatives, such as primary nursing, were virtually inevitable (Bowers 1989).

Besides possible improvements in patient care, the implementation of primary nursing is significant in terms of nurses' struggle to attain the status of professionals and to free nursing from the shadow of medicine. As Bowers (1989, p.15) puts it:

> primary nursing can be seen as part of nursing's search for identity, status and power. It appears to promise nurses the chance to work as individual practitioners in their own right, taking decisions about their own clients independently. It offers each nurse a degree of ability to control her own work ... It gives a rather different format for the relationship between doctors and nurses, indicating that it should be one of partnership rather than dominance/deference. A very rosy picture indeed, which makes the implementation of primary nursing seem both easy and very popular with nurses.

Yet interest in initiatives such as primary nursing has not only come from nurses: such developments have been significantly influenced by wider social and political forces. The Griffiths reorganisation has had a huge impact on the ethos of nursing and may help to explain the extent of support – for example, government funding to pilot Nursing Development Units – made available for initiatives such as the introduction of primary nursing. According to Bowers (1989, p.16), there are clear parallels between the organisational features of primary nursing and general management in the NHS:

> Areas of responsibility are clearly described, in that the primary nurse is responsible for her patients. The charge nurse/ward sister fulfils the role of ward general manager. Primary nursing provides at ward level a miniature reflection of general management in the NHS.

The notions of responsibility and accountability that are central to new nursing initiatives can also be seen as highly compatible with government priorities concerning management within the public sector (Bowers 1989). It is, then, for a variety of reasons that nursing and, within it, the nurse–patient relationship have come to be redefined.

CONTINUITY OF CARE

At the centre of many recent changes in nursing is a commitment to continuity of care for a patient by a particular nurse. For example, the Audit Commission (1991), which examined the use of resources by nurse managers in acute general hospitals, emphasised the importance of continuity of care if nursing practice and nurses' job satisfaction were to improve. Similarly, the named nurse system, called for by the Patient's Charter, has been interpreted as recognising not only the value of nursing but also the need for continuity of care (Hancock 1992, Wright 1992).

This commitment to continuity of care is clearly expressed in 'the new nursing' (Salvage 1990) – typified by primary nursing – which explicitly aims to transform interaction between nurses and patients and to promote patients' participation in care. Underlying the 'new nursing' is a belief that the relationship between nurse and patient has the potential to be therapeutic and central to the process of recovery (see for example Meutzel 1988, Wright 1991 and contributors to McMahon and Pearson 1991). Moreover, nursing care is understood very largely in terms of the nature of support offered to patients. For instance, in a study exploring the views of nurses and patients on how nursing care is thought to have affected the welfare of patients in hospital, Ersser (1991, p.71) finds that:

> [the] nurses' references to support bear a close similarity to those made by patients about caring. Each group describes the ways in which the nurse who provides care and/or support conveys a *proximity* to the patient in a variety of ways. These include, for example, 'presence' through *close* or frequent contact, remaining with and being attentive to the patient and conveying an understanding of the patient's experience. (my emphasis)

The value of 'being with' the patient or providing an 'existential presence' has been noted by a range of nursing authors (for example Meutzel 1988, Benner and Wrubel 1989, Ersser 1991) as well as non-nurses. Campbell (1984), for instance, describes the companionship that nurses offer patients as a 'closeness' that is neither sexual in nature nor a deep personal friendship, but rather a bodily presence: 'it involves a "being with" and not just a "doing to".' However, it is perhaps among exponents of primary nursing that 'closeness' is most clearly articulated.

PRIMARY NURSING

The difficulties of defining primary nursing and the variety of forms it can take have been widely commented upon (Giovannetti 1986, Mead 1991). According to Manthey (1992, p.26), primary nursing is:

> a system for delivering nursing service that consists of four design elements: i) allocation and acceptance of individual responsibility for decision making to one individual; ii) assignments of daily care by case method; iii) direct person to person communication; and iv) one person operationally responsible for the quality of care administered to patients on a unit 24 hours a day, seven days a week.

Primary nursing also represents one example of an organisational mode in which communication with patients is viewed as a central and legitimate aspect of nurses' work (Pearson 1988).

It is not yet clear whether this relatively new form of nursing has become associated with improved nursing outcomes. Some studies suggest that primary nursing produces higher quality care, as determined by nurses (Manley 1988), improved job satisfaction for nurses (MacGuire 1991) or higher efficiency (Binnie 1987). However, evaluation of primary nursing has generally been inconclusive, partly because of difficulties in clearly distinguishing it from other organisational modes (Mead 1991). Similarly, the introduction of primary nursing is often accompanied by interest in a range of issues, such as the importance of increased patient involvement, which are not exclusive to any particular way of organising care (Ersser and Tutton 1991). Evaluation has, for the most part, been restricted to more quantitative forms of analysis using, for example, Qualpacs – the Quality of Patient Care Scale – or Nursing Audit (Phaneuf 1976). While many aspects of nursing lend themselves to quantification, there remain issues of central importance to nursing that are less amenable to measurement and, therefore, remain largely unexplored (Lawler 1991, MacGuire 1991). Booth and Davies (1991), for instance, note that quality care audit is not always sensitive to some of the less concrete aspects of primary nursing, such as the potential for in-depth knowledge of the patient or the nature of the nurse–patient relationship. In summary, primary nursing proves hard to evaluate because it resists definition and because of an over-reliance on quantitative methods of evaluation.

CLOSENESS

According to Pearson (1988), in his description of the work of the Burford and Oxford Nursing Development Units and the utilisation of primary nursing, nurses achieve successful outcomes through the establishment of 'close' relationships with their patients and by using this 'closeness' to therapeutic effect in a planned and systematic way. Significantly, 'closeness' is seen, at least in part, to develop from the carrying out of intimate activities, such as bathing, for a patient in the context of a continuing relationship. The 'basic' work of nursing, traditionally relinquished as nurses became more senior, is now seen to provide the opportunity for psychological 'closeness' or a meaningful relationship between nurse and patient that may hold therapeutic potential (Meutzel 1988, Pearson 1988, Wharton and Pearson 1988, McMahon 1991).

References to 'closeness' occur frequently in recent nursing literature, yet the notion of 'closeness' has remained largely unexplored. Before the advent of the 'new nursing', Peplau (1969) described what she called 'professional closeness'. This she saw as sharing some features with the physical closeness and interpersonal intimacy found in non-professional relationships, but with its focus *exclusively* on the interests and needs of the patient. In other words, unlike many social relationships, those characterised by professional closeness are asymmetrical or non-reciprocal. According to Peplau (1969, pp.348–9), professional closeness is demonstrated by the nurse who:

shows that she can *put herself aside* and can bring all of her capacities, talents and competencies to bear upon the life of another person to the end that that person will grow a little, learn something new, and in effect be strengthened in a favourable direction. (my emphasis)

The 'closeness' that Peplau refers to (p.352) is 'not so much a matter of being closer to the person who is ill, but rather one of being "closer to the truth" of that person's current dilemma'. Significantly, professional closeness requires a special kind of detachment, and it is through their 'professional school' that nurses learn to demonstrate concern, competence and interest, while maintaining an emotional distance from the patient.

The notion of 'professional closeness' that Peplau described in the 1960s is, thus, apparently concerned with the maintenance of detachment. More recently, however, an alternative view has developed, with the ideal nurse–patient relationship portrayed as one of mutuality or reciprocity. Meutzel (1988), for example, suggests that the components of the therapeutic relationship between nurse and patient are partnership, reciprocity and intimacy, with self-disclosure and the giving of support evident on both sides. This points to a far more complex relationship than before. As Meutzel (1988, pp.106–7) puts it:

'Being there' is that intangible and paradoxically difficult and very simple essence of the dimension of reciprocity and intimacy. It is simple because it is in the desire for closeness of the philanthropic vocation 'to help people', difficult because a closeness that is mutually beneficial in a therapeutic relationship requires mature confrontation by the nurse . . . of the vulnerability of her own humanness.

Others have also referred to the significance of reciprocity and self-disclosure in the nurse–patient relationship. In a study of nurses' accounts of how their relationships with patients developed, Morse (1991) notes that, despite advice to the contrary, nurses develop clear strategies to increase their involvement with patients, including the mutual sharing of personal information. May (1991) describes a number of elements that underpin nurses' accounts of involvement with patients, including 'reciprocity', in which both nurse and patient convey to each other aspects of their private character. May also shows the need to disentangle the two meanings of 'involvement', suggesting that it may refer both to a general quality of nursing practice and to personal attachments to specific patients. It was in this second sense, where there might be an overemphasis on reciprocity, that 'involvement' could be problematic, in that it might demand a major investment on the part of nurses to sustain some form of equilibrium between their institutional role and their personal aspirations about commitment to patients.

POSSIBLE IMPLICATIONS OF 'CLOSENESS'

It has been suggested that the development of a 'close' relationship between a nurse and patient is thought to bring about radical change in practice (Pearson 1988, p.6). However, if task allocation were associated with defending the nurse from anxiety, new organisational modes stressing continuity of care would seem to pose new, personal challenges for nurses. Smith (1992, pp.9–10), for example, suggests that the introduction of the nursing process:

> with its explicit commitment to the development of nurse–patient relationships, puts the nurse at risk of increasing her anxiety by removing the protection provided by task-orientated care.

With individualised nursing care (especially with primary nursing where the number of patients each nurse cares for is limited and time spent with each patient is maximised), a number of disadvantages have been posited. Nurses may become unclear about the boundaries of their work; not only may nurses and patients become emotionally involved but over-involvement may lead to disagreements among members of the nursing team (Bowers 1989). Alternatively, a relationship of any depth with a patient may be emotionally costly for the nurse concerned. Moreover, the fragmentation of the ward staff into a number of small teams, each responsible for the needs of specific individuals, may reduce group cohesion and limit the support available for nurses (Reed 1992).

A number of researchers have looked at the different levels at which nurses may operate within their work relationships and the extent to which nurses may become involved (Benner 1984, May 1991, Morse 1991, Ramos 1992). These sorts of study are helpful in conceptualising the range of relationships that may exist for nurses and the association between these and the experience or expertise of individual nurses. However, by concentrating exclusively on the nurse–patient encounter, this kind of approach tends to overlook the sources of stress that reside in the organisational context of any such encounter. It overlooks, for example, the impact of workplace organisation and ethos on nurse–patient interaction. Occupational culture may play a significant role in the extent to which communication with patients is defined as work (Melia 1981, Smith 1992) or in whether 'involvement' is seen as a key element of nursing work (Field 1984). As May (1990) has pointed out, one of the problems with defining nurse–patient interaction as a therapeutic instrument is that it lays any failure to create therapeutic relationships at the feet of *individual* nurses, and overlooks the *collective* nature of nursing work. Alternatively, there is little work that examines the significance of general resources, such as managerial support, ancillary services or nurse staffing levels, on the development of meaningful nurse–patient relationships.

SUMMARY

Underlying the introduction of new nursing initiatives such as primary nursing is the rationale that developing the potential of nurse–patient interaction leads to improvements in patient care and nurses' job satisfaction. These improvements are thought to occur essentially through the establishment of 'close' relationships between nurses and patients, with this 'closeness' subsequently used to therapeutic effect. This notion of 'closeness' has remained largely unexplored, but there is a widespread assumption in the literature that the fostering of 'closeness' marks a radical departure from the traditional nursing approach in which nurses retained an emotional distance from patients. At the same time, a range of studies points to the problems nurses experience with current nursing trends in which sustained nurse–patient interaction is promoted.

Reading the literature associated with the 'new nursing' thus raises a number of questions which formed the focus of this research, namely:

- How do nurses understand the notion of 'closeness'?
- In what form and to what extent does 'closeness' feature in nurses' practice?
- Do nurses need additional skills or support if they are to employ the 'new nursing' effectively *and* without great personal cost, given the way in which this form of nursing is based on 'close' relationships?

ENDNOTES

1 It is worth noting Chapman's (1983) critique of Menzies' (1970) work at this point, as this is relevant to the research findings presented later. Briefly, Chapman notes that Menzies studied nurses in isolation from social and cultural norms and that her analysis suggests that 'intrapsychic' processes determine nurses' behaviour and the structure of the organisation in which they work. Other occupational groups, such as doctors, and their effects on nursing structures and behaviours are not considered, nor is the unequal distribution of power and authority in the hospital context considered as an influence on nurses' behaviour.

3

The Study

The research took place over a one-year period and focused on two medical/surgical wards, both specialising in gastrointestinal disorders. These wards were located in different inner-city hospitals in the south of England. The hospitals were both governed by the same health authority but fell within different nurse management structures.

One location, referred to as Jones Ward, was a Nursing Development Unit (according to both self-definition and the current King's Fund criteria, see Appendix) where primary nursing had been adopted. Nurses on the other site, Smith Ward, employed patient allocation as an organisational mode. Both wards are described in more detail in Chapter 4.

METHODOLOGICAL ISSUES

The study was primarily concerned with aspects of nurse–patient interaction. Significantly, the term 'interaction' implies actual behaviour as opposed to attitudes and role definitions; it refers to what people do, rather than what they might wish to do or perceive themselves doing (Diers and Leonard 1966). It cannot be assumed that nurses' attitudes and beliefs about the nurse–patient relationship and their actual interactions with patients will always correspond. This suggested a broad research approach for the study, allowing both the observation of behaviour and the eliciting of attitudes and perceptions, in order to assess the degree to which these overlapped.

With its focus on the interface between nurse and patient, the study raised a number of methodological issues not dissimilar to those faced by Lawler (1991) in her research concerning the way in which nurses manage their intimacy with the patient's body. Lawler observed that the knowledge nurses accumulate has arisen from practical, professional experience and is difficult to articulate; exploring this knowledge base raises inherent theoretical and epistemological problems for which there can be no single research approach. For similar reasons, a number of approaches – all within a qualitative paradigm – were chosen for this study, which *collectively* helped to build an account of nurse–patient interaction. This pluralist approach is also intrinsic to the development of an ethnography.

An ethnography represents an attempt to develop an understanding of a local world:

> the ethnographer first describes the local world and then, even if he or she is interested in particular persons, gives primacy not to the subjective reality of a single invidual but to the social reality of a particular group. For the ethnographer the local world that encircles the group may be a village or a neighbourhood or even a social network. (Kleinman 1992, p.128)

It is now widely recognised that ethnography, with its emphasis on the holistic description and understanding of a local world, is a valuable research method for nurse researchers (James 1984, Aamodt 1991). Robinson and Strong (1990), for example, used an ethnographic approach for researching nursing policy issues through focusing on (p.9):

> the feel of personalities, relationships, emotions, language, politics, customs, the comedy and the pathos, the mundane and the exotic, the real and the formal structures, the actual and the claimed behaviour, the whole and not just the part.

However, Kleinman cautions that an ethnographic approach to the study of illness and care generally culminates in a *mini*ethnography rather than a full ethnography, in that it tends to deal with a relatively narrow spectrum of experience within a local world. The danger of this narrow focus is that it may undercut the very purpose of ethnography, namely contextual analysis (Kleinman 1992, p.133). This research aims to describe the context in which nurses provide nursing care. However, due to the relatively short period of data collection, it is better to view this as an ethnographic approach, rather than a full ethnography.

Under the umbrella of an ethnographic approach, the main methods employed were:

- overt participant observation of interaction between nurses and patients;
- semi-structured, in-depth, tape-recorded interviews with nurses;
- overt observation of activities on the ward;
- informal interviews with nurses' colleagues who were associated with either ward. These informants included senior nursing staff and clinical nurse teachers, medical staff (predominantly consultants) and other health workers, such as the ward pharmacist or occupational therapist.

Findings were then presented to nurses on each ward, to invite their participation in the interpretation of data.

PARTICIPANT OBSERVATION

Among researchers in general, there is a tendency to focus on one aspect of human experience, namely the verbal, at the expense of other channels, such as sound, touch or smell (Stoller 1989). These other channels, according to Kleinman (1992), are central to understanding the meanings of illness and care and can be studied through an ethnographic approach based on participant observation.

Participant observation, one of the central planks of an ethnographic approach and the kitemark of anthropology, is often seen as a way of exploring informants' perspectives with minimum imposition of the researcher's preconceived ideas (Sapsford and Abbott 1992). As Boyle (1991, p.277) suggests:

> The term *participant observation* suggests that the researcher is directly involved in the informant's life, observing and talking with people as he or she learns their view of reality. The end result is that participant observation allows the researcher to take a particular slice of behaviour and interpret it by putting it into context.

Overt observation reduces some of the ethical objections to this method, but the disadvantage of reactivity – the possibility that the researcher's presence and behaviour will alter the research situation – remains.

In this study, in addition to *observing* through participation – that is, watching nurse–patient interaction while I worked on the ward – I also wanted to *participate*, in the sense of trying to understand the nurse's relationship to a patient through bodily involvement and the use of senses other than sight. This approach was based on the assumption of a close connection between bodily experience in the everyday world and the conceptual. In this, as indicated earlier, I have been influenced by the work of Jackson, who learnt from his fieldwork among the Kuranko of Sierra Leone that (1989, p.135):

> to participate bodily in everyday practical tasks was a creative technique which often helped me grasp the *sense* of an activity by using my body as others did. This technique also helped me break my habit of seeking truth at the level of disembodied concepts and decontextualised sayings.

Similarly, Stoller (1989) has challenged what he calls the 'visualism' of most ethnographies and suggests that giving attention to data collected through all the senses will make ethnographic accounts more accessible and more faithful to the realities of the field. Bloch (1991) makes a similar plea in order to make a slightly different point: that giving a description of how things look, feel, smell and taste acts as a reminder that data arise from sources other than linear linguistic thought. However, this raises a problem of how non-linguistic knowledge can be transmitted to others; it may be learnt through the body, but there is then a requirement to translate it into a linear, linguistic form of knowledge in order to make it available to the researcher's audience.

Bloch (1991, p.194) admits that in his own work in Madagascar he has, until recently, dealt with the problem of providing accounts of Malagasy culture by seeking confirmation through informants' statements of those things he already knows to be 'right' through previous participant observation:

> Like other anthropologists, I then pretend that the linguistic confirmation of these understandings . . . are the *basis* of what I understand, but this is not really so. My knowledge was established prior to these linguistic confirmations.

This approach of using the researcher's lived experience as data seemed particularly appropriate for the study of an occupational group whose work is not only based on a holistic view of the patient's experience, including that of the body, but may also include physical intimacy with patients as an integral part of the giving of care.

I had only limited success in making use of participant observation in this 'radical empirical' way. This was partly because the extent of my participation was limited by ethical and legal considerations; as I had not practised as a nurse for some time, I restricted myself to those practical tasks that posed no risks to the patient. The other constraint was time: I was unable to undertake the kind of prolonged fieldwork that characterises orthodox anthropology and appears even more important with radical empiricism. Probably because of this, I do not feel that I fully experienced – or could make myself aware of – the range of sources of data that were available through non-linguistic means. Nonetheless, my understanding of the field did benefit from this approach. I became aware, for example, of how, without conscious intent, I learnt to use my body as other nurses did on the wards, adopting similar forms of stance. Similarly, the way in which I used touch became more central to my interaction with patients, in a way that I would have *thought* inappropriate prior to fieldwork. As a result, I began to focus on the ways in which nurses used their own bodies in creating a specific context for the care they provided, a context that allowed them to shape and clarify the nature of their relationships with patients.

SEMI-STRUCTURED INTERVIEWS

In addition to the use of participant observation, in-depth, semi-structured, tape-recorded interviews were conducted with a number of nurses on both wards. These generally took place on the ward, in either an empty office, an empty patient's cubicle or, occasionally, a store room or linen cupboard!

I initially planned to interview both qualified and student nurses, and subsequently carried out a number of interviews with students. Ultimately, however, I have concentrated on the interviews with permanent staff as it became evident that this was more appropriate; the support needs of students and the support mechanisms available to them appeared quite different to those of qualified staff, and there were not the resources to research both areas.

Nurses were recruited to the study in slightly different ways on the two wards, although in both cases the 'sample' was opportunistic. I wanted to talk to a range of nurses, from those who were newly qualified to the most senior. Nurses within this spectrum were recruited according to whether they were willing and available. On Smith Ward, the pressure of work meant that it was more difficult for nurses to commit themselves to an interview ranging from 45 minutes to two separate sessions of about one hour each. The disadvantage of this approach was that in interviewing those nurses who were most accessible, I ran the risk of ignoring a group of nurses whose relative inaccessibility might, in itself, have been meaningful.

Because of the different grading structures on the two wards, there was no attempt to 'match' informants on the two wards, nor even the total number of interviews for each ward. On Jones Ward, I interviewed 10 permanent members of staff, including the health-care assistant. On Smith Ward, where there was no health-care assistant at the time, I interviewed nine permanent nurses. On both wards, interviews varied in nature according to the dynamic that developed between myself and those interviewed, the respondent's perception of the study and the extent to which we had worked together prior to the interview. All informants were broadly similar in age and ethnic identity but came from a range of social backgrounds. It is interesting to note that, despite this heterogeneity, family influence was one of the most common reasons nurses had for entering nursing (Tables 1 and 2).

ETHICAL CONSIDERATIONS

Particular problems or conflicts of interest may arise where nurses become simultaneous clinicians and researchers (Raudonis 1992). During fieldwork relatively few problems emerged as a result of this dual role, largely, I believe, because my nursing role was only partial. All patients that I worked with were aware of my status as a researcher, and it became evident that they also viewed me as a rather inexperienced or relatively unskilled nurse. This was made most apparent when an elderly patient said to me on going home, 'Well goodbye my dear and thank you. I know you are going to make a very good nurse.' There were two ways in which I believe I gave this impression of being a novice, despite having trained

Table 1   Jones Ward informants: age, grade, social background and reasons for entering nursing

Age	Grade	Social background	Reasons for nursing
31	I	mo = housewife fa = unskilled chemical worker	Needed a job; practical and theoretical
28	F	mo = nurse fa = carpenter	Influence of mother; variety
22	D	mo = home help fa = retired	Working with people
33	I	mo = secretary fa = school teacher	Told not clever enough for university
24	D	mo = social worker fa = school director	Sister's influence; a way to leave home
30	E	mo = nurse fa = entrepreneur	Family pressure
28	F	mo = housewife fa = bank manager (retd)	Both sisters were nurses; idea of helping people
32	HCA	mo = cleaner fa = labour contractor	No previous job; satisfaction
31	D	mo = school teacher fa = engineer (retd)	Contact with people; less socially intrusive than medicine
32	G	mo = housewife fa = carpenter	Practical

mo = mother
fa   = father
HCA = health-care assistant

25 years ago. One was that patients observed how, for any technical procedure, I always sought another nurse. The other way, however, was more subtle and of inherent interest to the research: I realised that I had the stance, gestures and movement of a beginner, particularly when I started working on the ward. This reflected my initial lack of confidence and also came about because the kinds of stance I was used to adopting as a nurse were now no longer in currency, at least on the wards where I carried out the research.

Those patients I did not work with but who might have seen me on the ward were often uninformed about my role as a researcher. Because of the way in which the work was organised, I rarely had any contact with these patients, and thus consent was not usually an issue. However, I occasionally found myself feeling rather compromised. For instance, if a patient I did not know walked down the ward and was obviously unsteady on his feet, I felt impelled as a nurse to offer him my arm and escort him to

Table 2 Smith Ward informants: age, grade, social background and reasons for entering nursing

Age	Grade	Social background	Reasons for nursing
23	E	mo = school support worker fa = self-employed (sales)	Childhood experience and school job experience
32	F	mo = care assistant fa = auditor	Could not do medicine; sister's influence
28	E	mo = nurse fa = wine connoisseur	Family of nurses; worthwhile
23	E	mo = nurse fa = bus driver	A way to leave home
32	G	mo = housewife fa = painter/decorator	Expressive; humanistic
27	E	mo = secretary fa = forensic scientist	Job security; variety
33	F	mo = housewife fa = farmer	Good scope for working with people
22	D	mo = shop manager fa = marine engineer	School encouragement; active; working with people
27	D	mo = housewife fa = skilled worker (retd)	Need for new start; family influence (uncles/aunts)

mo = mother
fa = father

his destination. This might then mean helping him into bed, for example, or onto the lavatory. In this context, I was unambiguously acting as a nurse and not a researcher, yet I would feel awkward that the patient was not aware of my research remit.

The other conflict of interest concerned my relationship with the other nursing staff. As a result of using participant observation, the boundaries between nurse, researcher and individual were not always clear. Some relationships developed into friendships, and there came a point at which it was important to decide to what extent the content of that friendship became data. For example, one of the primary nurses – outside the environment of the ward but still in the context of the hospital – offered additional information concerning issues we had previously discussed during interviews; this I counted as additional data. However, there were other occasions, such as going for a drink after work, which greatly contributed to my understanding of a group of nurses and how they worked together, but which I excluded as data. This goes against the usual practice of many anthropologists who might view this kind of informal interaction as the key to understanding informants' world views. However, I felt that I did not have informed consent to carry out my research in this sort of context.

In terms of the ethics of the research relationship and the issue of reciprocity between the researcher and the researched, I should add that nurses from both wards were extremely helpful and supportive towards me. I hope that I have been able to repay them in small ways, but I am aware that I remain greatly indebted to them.

REFLEXIVITY

According to Sapsford and Abbott (1992), reflexivity – a turning back on the researcher as subject – is important for three reasons: it acts as a form of self-monitoring and helps to minimise errors; it represents a form of data analysis, that is a way of understanding the data; and it helps to show that interpretations of the data are reasonable ones.

It has been suggested that the nature and quality of social research findings are significantly influenced by the nature of the relationship between researcher and researched, and that the characteristics of this relationship need to be made explicit This is because it cannot be assumed that all such relationships are similar in nature across all studies, while understanding the form of the relationship is important in assessing what has been discovered (Berg and Smith 1988).

In an attempt to describe my relationship with my informants (nursing and non-nursing), I shall also include details about access to the research field at this point. My work title of 'Research Fellow' was a useful one, in that it made little reference to any recognisable point in the nursing hierarchy. Similarly, holding a joint appointment between the College of Nursing and Midwifery and the Directorate of Quality Assurance (and, within this Directorate, being identified with the Department of Nursing Research and Development) was advantageous in that I was not clearly identified with any single institution.

Access to Jones Ward was also made easy through colleagues who already had strong links with the ward. As a Nursing Development Unit, Jones Ward had attracted a number of researchers, and some of the ward's staff were also carrying out their own research projects there. Staff were highly receptive to researchers and were used to being the focus of investigation. However, previous research had rarely involved participant observation or the initial uncertainty of focus that is often attendant upon a highly qualititative approach.

Access to Smith Ward was straightforward, given that I had no previous connection with any of the staff. My initial impression was that nurses were unaccustomed to having researchers on the ward, but this was not so; there was a range of research projects being carried out that I gradually became aware of, but, again, none were highly qualitative in nature.

It was difficult on both wards to give a clear picture of the research that I was carrying out, or rather of how the information I collected would be drawn together to make a meaningful statement on completion. Nonetheless, nurses were extremely helpful in accommodating me, whether this was through helping me find someone to attach myself to during participant observation, giving general information about the ward and the hospital in which it was located, or helping to organise interviews.

On both wards, I introduced myself to staff as both a nurse and an anthropologist, stating that I had not practised as a nurse for many years. My loss of nursing skills was a source of anxiety for myself but was useful in my relationships with nurses during participant observation: being seen as a learner or as an 'extra pair of hands' helped, I believe, to make my presence less threatening and, therefore, to some extent helped to 'normalise' the research setting.

Acceptance was also made easier during participant observation (which preceded interviews) by the adoption of a uniform. As Hammersley and Atkinson have remarked (1983, p.79), forms of dress give messages about the position that the ethnographer seeks to maintain. I generally wore a uniform dress, similar to that worn by other nurses on the ward. On Jones Ward, a number of nurses wore trousers and tunics, and I initially wore the same, before I realised that on Smith Ward the majority of nurses wore dresses. I felt it was important to wear the same sort of uniform on both wards, so from fairly early on in the research wore a uniform dress. A further decision was also required regarding a belt. I noticed that most nurses did not wear belts, so, after an initial period of trying to appear 'correct', I also dispensed with this. Similarly, I experimented with accessories such as hospital badges, scissor chains and fobwatches, finally excluding all but a name badge, which identified me as a research nurse.

There are two further considerations regarding research relationships and acceptance in the field that I would note, although I am unsure what weight to give these. One is age; I was between 10 and 20 years older than my informants, something that I became aware of only rarely – for example, when I was struck by a young nurse's assurance in a difficult situation and my own lack of skills in that context.

Additionally, kneeling or squatting like other nurses played havoc with my knees, which would seize up or made ominous noises of complaint; the informal stance I noted among nurses was clearly, among other things, the posture of youth. I cannot comment on the influence my greater age might have had on the research relationship, except that, in some instances, it became clear that I had a broader experience of life, which was connected to age.

The second consideration is that of gender. The majority of informants were female, working in a female-dominated occupation and doing what is widely interpreted as 'women's work'. Given the emphasis I place on the role of lived experience in the collection of data, and the possibility that women's experience mediated by the body is different to that of men's (see for example Young 1990, Savage 1992), the focus of the research, which developed through participant observation, might well have shifted had I not been a woman.

Similarly, my relationship to informants might have been different were I not female. This possibility was clearest in my interviews with medical consultants, although these particular research relationships were additionally influenced by the fact that I was a nurse as well as a social researcher. For example, despite introducing myself by letter as Dr Savage (a practice I avoided with potential non-medical informants), one of the consultants asked during the course of an interview whether I knew of a suitable person to carry out a research project for him, someone, like me, with 'a bit of an academic background'. I imagine that my 10 year training as an academic might have seemed a little weightier had I not been a woman or a nurse.

A NOTE ON THE ANALYSIS OF DATA

As Hammersley and Atkinson (1983, p.174) point out:

> In ethnography the analysis of data is not a distinct stage of the research. It begins in the pre-fieldwork phase, in the formulation and clarification of research problems, and continues into the process of writing up. Formally, it starts to take shape in analytic notes and memoranda; informally, it is embodied in the ethnographer's ideas, hunches and emergent concepts. In this way the analysis of data feeds into the process of research design.

Participant observation in the present study began with little formal idea of what it was that I was looking for in nurse–patient interaction, although I kept in mind anecdotal evidence suggesting that there was less humour where primary nursing was employed. This was despite the fact that during my first session on Jones Ward (during the selection of wards, see Chapter 4), I became aware that humour was used a great deal, sometimes in quite surprising ways. For example, my research notes on this first day record:

> Young man (24 years) solicitor, post-op (excision of pilonidal sinus) looked rather overcome by close proximity and interest of us all [at handover]. Sympathetic laughter from nurses and 'X' [associate nurse] says, 'We'll be getting in there with you in a minute'. Moment of (surprised?) silence after this. Sensed it was viewed as rather risqué statement but responded to eventually by moderated laughter – at least from other nurses.

It turned out that this was not a particularly characteristic use of humour by nurses on the ward. Instead, humour was usually non-sexual – especially with male patients of an age similar to that of staff. However, the tendency to use humour in order to deal with potentially embarrassing or unusual situations was a striking feature of everyday interaction.

In addition, nurses' use of touch and the way they positioned themselves in relation to patients was so striking that these became immediate foci of the study. Following my first, exploratory visit to Jones Ward, my notes included the following observation regarding touch:

> Much use made of touch, particularly by 'X' handing over/attempting to incorporate patient's perspective into nursing information. Touching knee, foot, hand, shoulder, arm at various points in discussion – for example, when trying to inform new shift of patient's need for analgesia and simultaneously indicate to patient that [his] need was understood as legitimate. Touch used to soften what was being said *and* demonstrate empathy. 'Y' [primary nurse] also used touch during handover – that is, with patients she had not met before – but less than 'X'.

This frequent use of non-instrumental touch was not observed on other wards visited while deciding where to carry out the research, and I began to feel that this use of non-instrumental yet non-spontaneous touch could be seen as a tangible representation of the nursing ethos on Jones Ward and of its nurses' understanding of the nurse–patient relationship.

Similarly, nurses on this ward made specific use of body positioning – most noticeably during handovers, but also at other times – which was, again, expressive but not entirely spontaneous. On my first, exploratory visit, for example, I observed the following during the midday handover:

> Bedside handover of four patients by 'X' and another [student] nurse. 'X' sitting on bed, 'Y' squatting by bedside near patient's head, me standing if no room to do anything else – otherwise sitting on bed. Felt, apart from my own self-consciousness, there was a certain self-conciousness about these arrangements on part of staff and patients. Dealt with at least in one instance by humour [see episode described above].

These themes of humour, touch and positioning, the relationship between them and their role in nurse–patient interaction were ones that recurred throughout fieldwork on Jones Ward and consequently became central to the study. When differences emerged between the ways in which staff on the two wards employed humour, touch and body posture, I began to ask myself about the extent to which the manipulation of these forms of communication was linked to the two wards' different organisational modes and the nature of interaction (for example degrees of 'closeness') that these might prompt between nurses and patients. In this way, I came to ask informants about how and why they employed touch, humour and posture in their work.

Data were generated in a number of ways. First, there were data that arose in response to my focus on categories (such as 'closeness') that were evident in the nursing literature and which I sought to understand in the

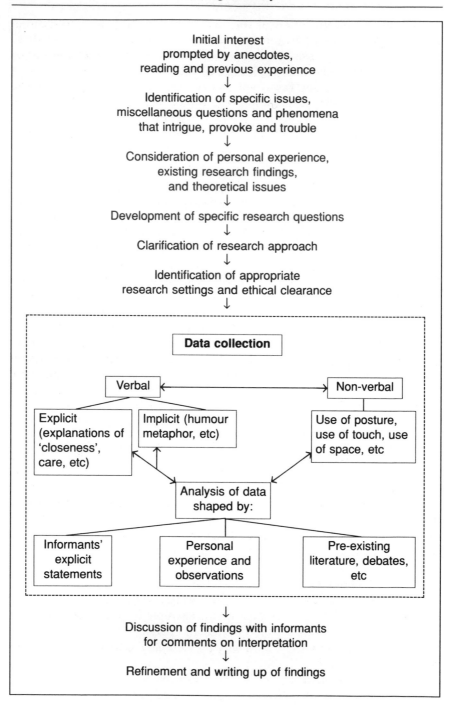

Figure 1   The research process

context of nursing practice. This involved my subjective interpretation of aspects of nurses' behaviour in addition to questioning nurses about these categories. Second, certain phenomena (such as nurses' use of posture or touch) became evident through participant observation, which again I asked nurses to consider but which I also interpreted in the context of the overall picture I was developing of the wards. Finally, a web of interconnected, *informant-generated* categories or notions emerged from nurses' interview transcripts, which I had not anticipated but which came to play an important role in understanding the data. These included the use nurses made of spatial metaphors, such as 'outside' and 'inside' – and, linked to this, 'going in' or 'getting right in' as a way of referring to the initial stages of involvement with a patient, the crossing of a boundary between the impersonal and the personal, or between distance and closeness. Other spatial metaphors that offered insights into nurses' perceptions of their interactions with patients included the significance of either party being 'open' or 'closed', the importance of 'lifting' patients who were 'down' and of 'getting down to the patient's level'.

These metaphors are further discussed in Chapter 8. Their relevance here is that, in common with many ethnographers, I utilise both *etic* and *emic* research styles (Robertson and Boyle 1984). In anthropology, emic analyses stress the subjective meanings shared by a social group together with their culturally specific 'model' of experience, while etic analyses involve the development of models derived from the analyst's theoretical categories. While some researchers concentrate on one approach or the other, or alternatively contrast the two approaches, it is increasingly recognised by anthropologists that a distinction between *emic* and *etic* is misguided. It fails to recognise that the researcher's own model is but another form of culturally specific 'model', informed by different meanings and experience but similarly subjective. On this basis, I have not refrained from interweaving my own analysis of the data with the perspectives made explicit by my informants. The overall process is represented in Figure 1. Similarly, the description of the two wards presented in the next chapter has been derived from both subjective and objective perspectives.

4

The Wards

THE CHOICE OF WARDS

The choice of wards was made after seeking advice about suitable locations from a range of nurses throughout the health authority, especially members of the local Nurses' Research Network. Eventually, six potential wards were identified, and the research was discussed with the senior staff of these units. A period of four hours was then spent on each ward as a participant observer in order to determine the most appropriate locations.

The main criterion for ward selection was that one ward should practise a form of nursing (such as primary nursing) in which the principles of the 'new nursing' could be identified, while the other ward should use a nursing mode that was less readily associated with this approach. Otherwise, the two wards should be as similar as possible with regard to variables such as specialty or sex of patients. A number of other factors had to kept in mind, however, such as the long-term plans for any ward or the number of other research projects already underway.

Eventually, it became clear that Jones Ward, with its commitment to primary nursing and its role as a Nursing Development Unit, represented the clearest example of the 'new nursing'. Smith Ward was then chosen because it shared the specialty of gastroenterology with Jones Ward and it employed a different organisational mode, namely patient allocation. The intention was not to compare wards in the sense that possible differences in nurse–patient interactions might be viewed as the result of different organisational modes; indeed, with the two wards finally chosen there were too many variables to make this a feasible proposition. Instead, I hoped to make use of my experience on each ward to sharpen my thinking about the other and to describe similarities and differences, which could then be explored.

JONES WARD

Jones Ward was a 17-bed, mixed medical and surgical ward for male patients. For the most part, patients had disorders of the gastrointestinal tract, particularly of the bile duct and pancreas. Generally, patients had relatively little need of physical nursing care but were often chronically unwell, and readmissions were common. Primary nursing had been in use for almost four years.

In addition to a senior nurse who covered the entire gastroenterology unit, of which this ward formed a part, there were three primary nurses employed on the ward, each with 24-hour accountability for a group of five to six patients from their admission to discharge. Primary nurses had five to eight years post-registration experience, although the formal prerequisite was two years. In the absence of the primary nurse, care was provided by an associate nurse, usually a D grade or student nurse, in accordance with the care plan. (For details of each ward's staff establishment, see Figures 2 and 4 below.) During the research period, student nurses were not supernumerary.

The form of nursing practised on Jones Ward conforms to Manthey's (1992) definition of primary nursing (see Chapter 2), but it would have been classified as a variant of team nursing if Thomas and Bond's (1990) questionnaire had been used to determine the organisational mode. For example, with only three primary nurses, it was not possible for each, as care planner, to give continuity of care. Thus, care was shared within three groups of nurses on the ward, each 'headed' by a primary nurse. This discrepancy between Manthey's and Thomas and Bond's classifications is interesting, as it helps to highlight just how broad a concept primary nursing can be and how difficult it is to define. In addition to following Manthey's principles in organising care, nursing practice on Jones Ward

Official establishment	Actual establishment
	1 G grade nurse
3 F grade nurses	2 F grade nurses
	1 E grade nurse
7 D grade nurses	6 D grade nurses
1 Health-care assistant	1 Health-care assistant

Additional staff with clinical involvement

1 I grade senior nurse (with responsibility for entire GI unit)
1 I grade nursing development facilitator

Figure 2 Establishment of permanent staff for Jones Ward during the study

was guided by a concept of 'partnership with the patient' that implied a non-authoritarian relationship and an emphasis on communication between nurses and patients. Primary nursing for nurses on Jones Ward was, therefore, not merely an organisational mode, but also a philosophy of care. In many ways (and partly because of the commitment to peers that existed among its nurses), nursing on Jones Ward went a long way towards Meutzel's description of 'renaissance nursing' as not simply a 40-hours-a-week job, but a 24-hours-a-day commitment.

Walking onto Jones Ward, I was often struck by its sense of light and space, and its peaceful atmosphere. The perception of light and spaciousness came from the ward layout. The ward was of Nightingale design with a high ceiling and many tall windows on two sides of the ward. Most of the beds were spaced well apart. Yet, perhaps the greatest contribution to the sense of spaciousness was the absence of any nursing station on the ward; there was simply a very small desk for a telephone in the centre of the ward.

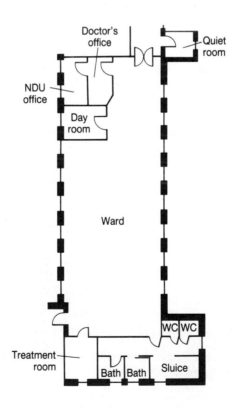

Figure 3 Layout of Jones Ward

The peaceful atmosphere was the result of a number of factors. There was no Accident and Emergency (A&E) department at the hospital, so emergency admissions of acutely ill patients were rare. The lack of emergency admissions meant that the vast majority of patients came under the auspices of only three consultants, those with specified beds on the ward. Thus, doctors and medical students visiting the ward were restricted to three 'firms', and, even for these, teaching rounds with large entourages of medical students were uncommon. 'Traffic' was also reduced on the ward because many patients were fairly mobile and did not, for example, require porters with wheelchairs in order to attend other departments for treatments or investigations. Additionally, those patients who were well enough would wander off to the hospital garden or shop, or to the stairwell outside the ward, often to smoke. The ward was, therefore, often half empty of its residents.

Beyond these factors, much of the atmosphere of the ward was formed by the way in which nurses carried out their nursing activities. Although a mixed medical and surgical ward, only a minority of Jones Ward's patients underwent major surgery. Most procedures were relatively minor, such as scans or endoscopies. Nurses, therefore, did not move briskly as they tend to on busy surgical wards. Instead, much of the nurses' time was spent sitting with patients or relatives; this was seen as a central element of nursing care, irrespective of the need for practical procedures. Nurses were able to spend time with patients largely because staffing levels were good and hospital resources were such that nurses did not generally feel obliged to take on non-nursing duties. In addition, they had organised their work in order to meet their priority of 'spending time with patients' through, for example, removing any central nursing station; this meant that all paperwork was carried out at the bedside.

Nurses on Jones Ward also made what seemed to be a deliberate use of their body, consciously sitting or squatting by their patients, rather than standing over them during any interaction. As a result, the scene at times was more domestic than institutional and more reminiscent of a private sitting room than part of a hospital. The nature of care on the ward was characterised by the health-care assistant who said:

> It's not so physically demanding on this ward as, I'd say, compared to a busy care of the elderly ward. It can be mentally quite tiring and quite stressful working on this ward sometimes; the majority of patients are very ill, and the majority of your time is spent sitting down talking to them about their problems or any fears they've got and just trying to reassure them.

SMITH WARD

Smith Ward was located in a different hospital within the health authority and was subject to different management styles and levels of resources. It was, at the outset of the study, a 24-bed, mixed medical and surgical ward, comprising four bays and six cubicles, although one of these was converted to a store room during the research period in an attempt to lighten the nursing workload.

Most patients on Smith Ward, both male and female, had disorders of the gastrointestinal tract, many of which were malignant. However, five of the beds were allocated to patients who were admitted for palliative laser treatment of œsophageal lesions. These patients might be terminally ill and highly dependent on nursing care. Besides this group, a significant proportion of the 'GI' patients were elderly, not very mobile and perhaps doubly incontinent. There were, thus, heavy demands on staff for 'basic' nursing care.

Patient allocation was in use as an organisational mode when the research project began, although team nursing was later introduced as it was seen to offer a means of putting the named nurse concept into practice. In terms of nursing philosophy, there were similarities with Jones Ward; for example, nurses subscribed to the view that the nurse–patient relationship should, as far as possible, be one of equality, and that nurses should act as the patient's advocate if necessary. These similarities existed despite the retention on Smith Ward of a more traditional organisational mode and grade mix.

The ward had a more traditional staffing structure than Jones Ward (Figure 4), with a Charge Nurse in overall charge of the ward (under the patient allocation regime), supported by two senior (F Grade) staff nurses in addition to a number of E and D grade staff nurses. There was no health-care assistant at the time of the study, and student nurses still formed a central component of the workforce.

One of the strongest impressions I had, walking onto Smith Ward, was of entering a rabbit warren or even an ant colony (Figure 5). It was relatively dark and there was no sense of space or of peace. Emergency admissions from A&E meant that the beds were used by a large number of medical and surgical firms. Thus, the number of junior house officers on the ward was relatively high. Consultant and teaching rounds were

---

1 G Grade nurse
2 F Grade nurses
6 E Grade nurses
6 D Grade nurses

2 D grade posts were frozen during the study

Figure 4 Establishment of permanent staff for Smith Ward during the study

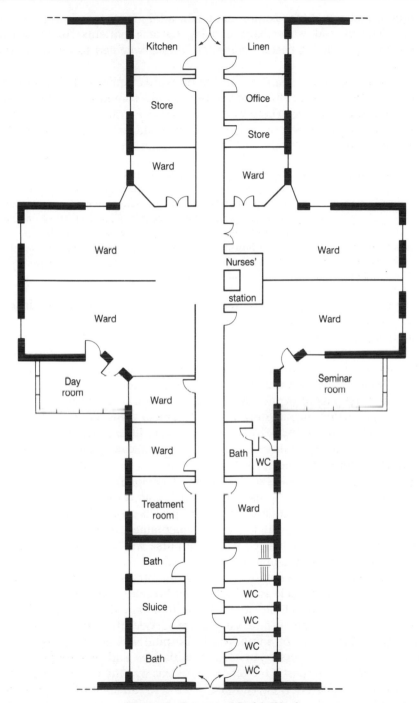

Figure 5 Layout of Smith Ward

frequent and sometimes conterminous. In addition, there always seemed to be trolleys and wheelchairs arriving to take patients for investigations and procedures, besides commodes being wheeled to and from the sluice.

Generally speaking, patients on Smith Ward required skilled surgical nursing with a view to their early return to the community, or palliative care for terminal illness. There were few long-stay patients, and these were often awaiting the action of the Social Services department. As one senior staff nurse said:

> On this ward, because there's such a cross-section of patients . . . laser patients at times tend to be like hospice patients, there's that aspect of it, then on the other aspect you've got surgical patients who are having active, aggressive treatment . . . I've never been in a situation where there's been such a contrast of patients. It causes quite an antagonism between the two – how you care for the one and how you care for the other. I find it quite a demanding place to give a level of care I would consider acceptable. Even over the past three years, it's [become] more difficult to meet an acceptable standard.

In this last sentence, the nurse refers to a range of changes experienced over recent years, ranging from a faster turnover of patients to chronic understaffing, resulting, in part, from the freezing of two D grade posts.

While nurses placed great emphasis on the importance of talking to patients, I did not often observe nurses sitting with patients, as I had on Jones Ward. There were a number of reasons for this. To begin with, because of the layout of the ward, it was more difficult to observe nurse–patient interaction overall, only a limited number of incidents occurring in one part of the ward. In addition, there was very little space between beds. For example, except for those in the ward cubicles, each patient's space was seriously reduced by the arrival of their neighbour's visitors. The close proximity of others made the discussion of personal issues very difficult. Moreover, a great part of nurses' time was required for instrumental care; the time available for patients not requiring such care was limited, and, of necessity, interaction might be largely maintained in passing: greetings and quips would be exchanged while the nurse was en route to someone else. Lack of time resulted partly from the nature and pace of work on the ward and the shortage of staff, and also from nurses' greater involvement in non-nursing duties due to a shortfall in hospital support services. For example, at the time of the study, I was told that there were only five porters to cover all the hospital's in-patient services. In addition, the nurse management structure of Smith Ward's hospital was perceived by nurses of both hospitals as less open to new initiatives and less supportive to staff than its counterpart. One reflection of this was the different opportunity for post-registration education available to nurses on the two wards (Table 3).

Table 3   Differences in post-registration training/education between the two wards

	Jones Ward	Smith Ward
Degrees prior to nursing	1 (psychology)	–
Degrees since training	–	1 (sociology) [full time]
Professional courses	ENB 100 (1)	B Tech (2)
	RCNT (1)	
	ENB 870 (2)	
Currently studying	Diploma in Nursing (1)	–
	BSc Health Studies (1)	
	BSc Nursing Studies (1)	
Future studies	MSc	Care of the dying
	(medical anthropology)	

DIFFERENCES AND SIMILARITIES BETWEEN NURSING TEAMS

There were subtle differences between the wards in relation to the nurses who were interviewed. Of course, the study deals with very small numbers of staff, so no claim can be made for statistically significant findings. Instead, features of the ward teams which might have some bearing on the way they conceptualise and practise nursing are described (Tables 4 and 5). Broadly speaking, nurses' ages, socioeconomic background (as indicated by education prior to nursing and parental occupations) and social class (self-defined) were broadly similar for nurses on both wards. Similarly, there were no enormous differences in terms of nurses' reasons for entering nursing or in their interests, as gauged by their television, newspaper or nursing journal habits. There was some difference in that on Jones Ward more nurses interviewed came originally from London and the Home Counties, while nurses interviewed on Smith Ward more often came from the north of England, Scotland, Northern Ireland and Eire. There was also a slight difference in terms of religion. Nurses interviewed on Smith Ward were more likely than those on Jones Ward to describe themselves as 'religious' or to have strong opinions about belief systems. The possible relevance of any differences between ward teams is considered in Chapters 6 and 9.

INTERPERSONAL RELATIONSHIPS AMONG STAFF

Several of the nurses on Jones Ward had worked together for over four years and, as a group, had experienced a number of changes, such as the relocation of the ward and a new specialty (previously it was haematology) and organisational mode. Not surprisingly, perhaps, there was a core group of nurses who shared a relatively long social history as well as an occupational

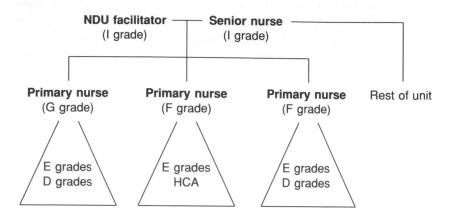

Figure 6   Flattened hierarchy: Jones Ward

Table 4   Informants' reading and viewing habits, regional and religious backgrounds: Jones Ward

Place of upbringing	Religious background	Reading and viewing habits	
Rochdale	Lapsed Roman Catholic	*Guardian*	Soaps, documentaries
North Wales/Chester	Christian	*Independent*, *Telegraph*	Soaps, documentaries, wildlife
Chelmsford	Christian	–	Soaps, mystery
Hertfordshire/Devon	–	*Guardian*, *Observer*	Soaps, news, films, plays
Belfast	Roman Catholic	–	Soaps
Inner London	–	*Independent*	'Anything'
London, Kent, Sussex	–	*Daily Mail*	Wildlife, mystery
Inner London	–	*Independent*, *Guardian*	Films, documentaries
Cornwall, Nottingham	–	–	News
Surrey, Kent	Church of England	–	Films

Table 5 Informants' reading and viewing habits, regional and religious backgrounds: Smith Ward

Place of upbringing	Religious background	Reading and viewing habits	
Cheshire	Lapsed United Reformed	*Independent*	News, soaps
Doncaster, Yorkshire	Church of England	*Telegraph, Independent*	Soaps, documentaries
Jersey, Derby	Church of England	*Daily Mirror*	Soaps
Inverness	Agnostic	*Daily Mirror*	Soaps
Eire	Roman Catholic	Assorted	Documentaries
Bristol, Birmingham, Solihull	–	*Guardian*	News, documentaries
Eire	Roman Catholic	*Times*	Documentaries
Scotland	Born-again Christian	*Glasgow Herald, Scotsman*	Soaps, mystery, documentaries
Northern Ireland	Quasi-Spiritualist	Tabloids	Soaps, arts

one. This group consisted predominantly, but not entirely, of the more senior nurses on the ward. It was my impression that it was these nurses, for the most part, who were the proselytisers of primary nursing and the most innovative among the overall team in terms of developing nursing practice on the ward. At the same time – and paradoxically, given the assumptions about the egalitarian nature of primary nursing – this group could be seen to represent a level of 'flattened' hierarchy (Figure 6); they appeared to be the collective holders of power within a wider group that was committed to equality, at least in the nurse–patient relationship. This impression of hierarchy was supported by the comments of one of the more senior nurses, for example, who observed how associate nurses often appeared inhibited in their contributions to ward meetings. Yet wherever the locus of power lay, it was clear from nurses' accounts that they received support from across the range of ward staff (see Chapter 9), and most students and associate nurses spoke in a highly positive way about their ward experience.

The relation between ward nurses and medical staff was also difficult to characterise. The ideology informing the practice of primary nursing stresses the distinctiveness of nurses' knowledge and the autonomy of nursing practice. Thus, in theory, primary nursing represents a challenge to the traditionally hierarchical relationship between medical and nursing staff. On Jones Ward, this challenge was apparent in some areas of practice but not in others. The relationship between nurses and junior doctors generally appeared convivial, although as a participant observer I was struck by a sense of invisibility in exchanges with medical staff. Particularly in the case of senior doctors, nurses did not appear to be recognised as individuals. For example, I observed one consultant enter the ward, greeting the nurses with a cry of, 'Morning, girls', apparently blind to both the range of ages among female nurses and the presence of male student nurses. Such invisibility would seem unlikely were there a relationship of equality between nurses and doctors.

At least one consultant suggested that all was not well between the nursing and medical staff, believing that most doctors experienced difficulties working on the ward, stemming from the assertiveness of some nurses. This consultant's impression, however, was in part formed as a result of information fed to him via a third party who, it has to be noted, had a strong antipathy to primary nursing and, apparently, to the nursing staff on Jones Ward. It was clear, however, that there was general dissatisfaction among medical staff regarding the way in which ward rounds were accompanied by a sequence of different – and often junior – nurses and that doctors had to seek out the appropriate nurse for a particular patient. According to one consultant, dealing with the nurse who was the direct care-giver did not lead to enhanced information about patients, only the wrong sort of information; nurses were seen to emphasise how patients were *feeling* when what was required were 'facts'. There was a sense, then, that nurses and doctors were operating within different paradigms, that nursing knowledge had changed and that nurses' perspectives of patients' needs had shifted away from those of doctors.

Significantly, if the knowledge that nurses drew upon had undergone a shift of paradigm, there was little corresponding shift in the power that was available to nurses. As one student nurse said of Jones Ward, for example:

> It's very consultant-based; what [the consultant] says goes. I've been used to dressing operation sites and for the wound – if it's not oozing – to be open. Here dressings stay; [you] don't touch a dressing unless you're told by a doctor, and I feel you've really gone back to being a handmaiden on this ward. You're doing what the doctor's ordering. Your initiative's really taken away from you.

Nurses' relationships with non-medical staff appeared very different from those with doctors. For example, the ward pharmacist had a clear understanding of the nursing ethos on Jones Ward and recognised that her own manner on the ward had been positively influenced by this. She recalled, for example, how with one patient who was blind, she had taken to sitting on his bed and holding his hand while explaining his medications.

This, she felt, was an approach she had learnt from ward staff. With one or two exceptions, nurses on Jones Ward had good relations with other nurses in the hospital, although I believe they were seen to be out of touch with the broad realities of nursing by at least some nurses in other hospitals in the group.

If they had previously been unaware of them, these realities increasingly came to bear on the everyday life of Jones Ward staff. Despite having a very clear idea of the kind of nursing they wanted to practise, nurses, over the research period, appeared to experience a loss of direction. This seemed to stem from changes among staff, from the long-term difficulties of continuing and sustaining change, from difficulties with future funding and from broader influences beyond the ward. The ward facilitator, who was central to the development of nursing practice, was funded by 'soft money', and her future was becoming uncertain. In addition, both hospitals were facing the prospect of cuts in services and staff and both wards were at risk of closure or significant change beyond their control. Shortly after my period of fieldwork, it became clear that Jones Ward was to be relocated and amalgamated with other wards. After 18 months of uncertainty, Smith Ward was relocated to another hospital.

Smith Ward, like Jones Ward, had been very stable in terms of staff turnover. Similarly, some nurses would socialise together after work. What was different was that on Smith Ward, all nurses on the same shift would come together as a group for the handover and, in the case of the late shift, for the tea break. The majority of nurses – a group that appeared roughly to correspond with those who smoked – used the charge nurse's office for breaks. This was in contrast to nurses on Jones Ward who, if they stayed near the clinical area for their break, used a room which was shared with staff on the adjacent ward; there was no specific time or space in which the group identity of the ward's nurses might be routinely consolidated or reinforced. Although there was a great deal of joking on both wards between nurses, the sense of a unified team was more apparent on Smith Ward, at least to outsiders. As one consultant on Smith Ward said of the ambiance created by nurses, 'It's very much a family affair'. Morale was seen to be good by the nurse manager and by medical colleagues, although many nurses privately expressed their anger about the lack of resources available to them and their patients, together with their anxieties about the future.

Among doctors and nurses within and beyond the hospital, Smith Ward had a high reputation for the standard of nursing it offered. The senior staff were seen to provide excellent role models. Reference was made to the flexibility of the ward team and to their skills in getting at the root of patients' problems. Some praise was qualified; nurses did a good job 'under the circumstances' – referring, for example, to the difficulties imposed by the ward's layout and decrepitude. A number of doctors and other colleagues were aware of the difficulties of providing good care where there was a mix of short-stay patients requiring palliative care, surgical patients requiring preparation and post-operative care, and medical patients who were perhaps relatively long-stay and heavily dependent on physical nursing care.

As with Jones Ward, relationships with junior doctors were generally cordial. On Smith Ward, however, not only were there more doctors to be seen on the ward, but also they seemed to spend longer periods of time on the premises. However, while they might congregate around the nurses' station, they generally interacted more with other doctors than with nurses. The charge nurse told me how some male junior doctors had complained that nurses on Smith Ward did not flirt like others in the hospital.

Senior doctors had other complaints, remarking on the way that nurses did not seem to know about all the patients on the ward, and saw this as poor nursing practice. There was a confusion in doctors' minds between levels of communication between nurses and doctors on the one hand and nursing care on the other. One consultant, despite praising Smith Ward as one of the best organised wards in the hospital, had a low opinion of nursing in general, believing it to have declined in quality over the previous 10 years or so. He felt that nurses were less dedicated, had less knowledge (implicitly, quasi-medical knowledge) than previously and tended to excuse their lack of knowledge about a specific patient by referring doctors to other nurses, saying, '[He or she] is not my patient'.

It was also suggested by medical colleagues that wards were more dirty and untidy than in the past, with the implication that nurses were accountable for this decline. This view was commented on spontaneously by the charge nurse on Smith Ward who said:

> There's this 'housekeeping' attitude [doctors] tend to have towards sisters and charge nurses. For example, '[charge nurse], we've run out of such and such; could you make sure we have it next time?' or, 'Goodness me, this ward is extrememly untidy' . . . 'It's not very clean'. And I say, 'Well, I didn't train as a domestic' and, 'I'd have it taken up with the domestic supervisor – could you refer it to them please?'

Patient allocation might be seen as more traditional than some other organisational modes, and features of traditional nursing, such as the attendance of the ward coordinator (often the most senior nurse on duty) throughout each consultant ward round, were evident on Smith Ward. However, the power dynamic between nurses and doctors was clearly of concern to nurses. The charge nurse said, for example:

> You know, [there's] this constant *unwillingness*, I think, on doctors' part to allow nurses to assume any position of power.

His perception of the power relations may have been heightened by virtue of being a man in what is widely assumed to be an occupation for women. There was, however, a questioning attitude among many of the ward's nurses which meant that issues of power were recognised and articulated. This questioning attitude also played a role in the ward's retention of patient allocation; there was a reluctance to 'jump on the band wagon' and adopt a new form of organisational mode where it might be inappropriate. Patient allocation was seen as a legitimate way of solving some of the problems that were specific to Smith Ward, such as the difficulties posed for continuity of care by the combination of its geographical layout and sex mix of patients; it was feared that these difficulties would be tackled less effectively by other organisational modes.

Within the nursing team, there was a conventional mix of grades (Figure 7), and the charge nurse was said, by a number of informants, to like to 'hold the reins'. In addition, on each shift the activities of the team were facilitated by a nurse coordinator, who was generally the most senior nurse on duty. However, the remaining nurses of all grades were either allocated or chose a number of patients each and were then responsible for the care of these specific patients. Thus, nurses, even quite junior nurses, had a fairly high degree of autonomy in terms of the care they gave individual patients, compared with, for example, their peers on wards where primary nursing was employed. There, it seemed that the primary nurse, even when not directly giving care, retained prime responsibility for planning care.

Nurses' autonomy on Smith Ward was evident at another level. Across grades, nurses were generally articulate in discussions with other team members in a way that was often referred to as 'bluntness'. As the charge nurse commented:

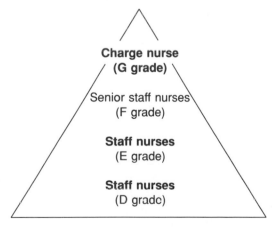

Figure 7 Traditional hierarchy: Smith Ward

I think a lot of us – we're very *earthy* people, you know. Pragmatic. Practical. It tends to be informal, but it can also be a bit abrasive at the same time.

This perception of the ward team as pragmatic was shared by other nurses I spoke to on Smith Ward and contrasted with the 'vision' of nurses on Jones Ward. It is this contrast of emphasis – the pragmatic versus the visionary – which is further discussed in Chapter 9, that appears to lie at the heart of any difference between the two wards. Yet as we shall begin to see in the following chapter in which nurses' views on the various organisational modes are presented, any difference in emphasis appeared to be strongly linked to the local conditions faced by nurses, rather than to reflect an essential difference in their philosophy of care.

5

Nurses' Perceptions of Organisational modes

There are a number of ways of organising nursing care for patients and much debate about which is the most appropriate in any setting to promote continuity of care. Nurses on both wards in this study were asked for their views on the organisational modes of primary nursing, team nursing and patient allocation. The majority of nurses on Jones Ward had had experience of all three different ways of delivering care at some point in their nursing careers. On Smith Ward, only a minority of nurses interviewed had previously worked in a context in which primary nursing was employed.

There were two reasons for asking nurses about these ways of delivering care. The first was to clarify how nurses in the study understood these organisational modes, given, for example, the variety of ways in which these can be interpreted (see for example Giovannetti 1986 on primary nursing) and the way in which local conditions might constrain the implementation of certain modes in their ideal form. Also, nurses' comments concerning these modes of organisation might say something about their perceptions of the notion of 'care' or their priorities regarding the giving of care. A brief description of the features of these organisational modes, taken from orthodox nursing discourse, is provided at the beginning of each section below. This is offered for those readers who are unfamiliar with systems for delivering nursing care and to provide a backdrop to what nurses from Smith or Jones Wards have to say regarding their own experience of these systems.

PERCEPTIONS OF PRIMARY NURSING

Primary nursing is described as a professional model of practice, in which a
qualified nurse is responsible and accountable for the nursing care of a case
load of patients, for the entire duration of their care in that particular setting
(eg ward, group home, own home). The principles of primary nursing are:

- The allocation and acceptance of individual responsibility and accountability for decision making to one individual nurse.
- Assignments of daily care, ie the individual receiving total care from
  one nurse, who has the freedom to carry out this practice (autonomy).
- Direct person to person communication.
- One nurse responsible for the co-ordination and quality of care admin-
  istered to a group of patients 24 hours a day, 7 days a week.

The values underpinning primary nursing centre on the belief that the
nurse–patient relationship is therapeutic. It provides an environment
and philosophy in which nurses can achieve their maximum potential in
patient centred care.

(Royal College of Nursing 1992a)

The vast majority of nurses interviewed on Jones Ward (including non-
permanent staff) were in favour of primary nursing. Primary nursing was
seen, more than team nursing or patient allocation, to allow continuity of
care, which was highly prized. Nurses appreciated not being moved from
group to group, as might happen elsewhere when staff shortages occurred.
Nurses also thought that with primary nursing they tended to nurse fewer
patients. This led to greater job satisfaction and the sense of working as an
independent practitioner, because of being able to carry through all aspects
of care.

The most commonly expressed advantage of the system, however, was
that primary nursing allowed nurses to get to know their patients better, to
establish better relationships and to communicate more effectively with
their patients. For example, one associate nurse said of primary nursing on
Jones Ward:

Here you definitely know your patients very well; you know what is happening.
You build up quite a good relationship. I guess you could get more attached to
them.

One primary nurse described this aspect of primary nursing with explicit
reference to 'closeness', saying:

The difference is you get to know patients and their families much better . . . there is a much closer relationship, particularly when they come in repeatedly. And it tends to be easier to spot the little things that might have gone unnoticed before, because you know the person that much more closely; you can spot things that maybe you wouldn't if you didn't know them so well.

While primary nurses clearly felt that they had greater accountability and responsibility, the experience of more junior nurses was less uniform. Some nurses valued the opportunity of being the only nurse on duty for a patient group during a shift, but at least one student nurse felt restricted by being unable to alter care plans without conferring with the primary nurse and enjoyed the freedom brought by night duty, when there were generally two nurses covering the entire ward. This student also felt that continuity of care led to lack of variety. She thought that the emphasis on 'talking with patients' often meant that conversations became unspontaneous once certain subjects had been explored:

When you keep seeing the same faces . . . you do run out of things to say to a patient. You know, you can talk about the weather and Christmas, but then you feel you're really forcing yourself to make conversation.

However, other staff appeared to interpret 'talking to patients' in a different way, namely as an opportunity to look at a wide variety of a patient's needs. For example:

Sometimes we're very busy on [Jones], but the majority of the time we can spend more time actually sitting down talking to the patient dealing with psychological needs, instead of just physical needs. (Health-care assistant)

Most nurses expressed some concern about the way in which the division of patients and nurses into three exclusive groups tended to fragment the ward team. This posed the risk of poor communication between groups and the threat of an overall loss of team spirit. Initially, nurses found it difficult to adjust to this aspect of the system, and felt uneasy that they did not have an overview of what was happening on the ward. This (as suggested in Chapter 4) was particularly difficult in terms of relationships with non-nursing colleagues, especially in relation to ward rounds with doctors. These brought more junior nurses into contact with senior medical staff and created difficulties for some nurses who felt unconfident or intimidated in this role.

Nurses on Smith Ward generally had little experience of primary nursing. One senior staff nurse had worked on a ward during the implementation of primary nursing and, after the teething problems, felt that 'they got it running very, very well'. However, she thought that the way it was organised was steeply hierarchical, with responsibility and skills retained by a few key members of the ward staff.

PERCEPTIONS OF TEAM NURSING

> Team nursing is based on the belief that a small group of nurses working together, led by one nurse, can give better care than they can if they work individually. It uses the skills of all team members so that the client gets the best care available. This small team is responsible and accountable for their group of patients during the whole of the patient's hospital stay.
>
> There are 3 prerequisites for team nursing:
>
> - Each team is led by a registered nurse, who must have leadership and management skills.
> - There must be effective written and spoken communication.
> - The style of management must support the role of the team leader.
>
> There are a number of ways the team can choose to organise their client's care on a daily basis, and there is flexibility in the size of the team, the case load, and the time span of each case load.
>
> (Royal College of Nursing 1992a)

Most nurses on Jones Ward had previously had good experience of team nursing but felt that, as an organisational mode, it did not allow the same continuity of care as primary nursing. This was largely because the number of patients cared for by a team (usually about 12) meant that nurses moved more between patients. Consequently, they felt nurses using this mode did not get to know their patients as well. For example:

> [Team and primary nursing] are fairly similar to a degree, but the number of patients you have is slightly larger with team nursing, so you don't always get the same patients again; there's not always continuity. You might not get to know your patients in quite so much depth. (Associate nurse)

Some perceptions of team nursing, however, were influenced by chronic understaffing, which made continuity of care even more difficult to achieve.

One of the clearest distinctions drawn between team and primary nursing was that the role of the team leader was seen to be different from that of the primary nurse: the team leader was not necessarily a care-giver and was thus not accountable for every patient allocated to the team. Only one nurse on Jones Ward – a student – preferred team nursing to primary nursing, largely because she felt that nurses had a better overview of the ward.

A number of nurses on Smith Ward had experience of team nursing. Several felt ambivalent about this organisational mode. Team nursing was seen to hold potential benefits for patients in that 'they get more sense of belonging and continuity'. It was seen to allow nurses the possibility of forward planning as well as the satisfaction of continuity of care. However, team nursing was seen as vulnerable to collapse where there were shortages of staff, and, importantly, continuity of care was not always seen in entirely positive terms. Moreover, when it was not properly implemented, team nursing could have a divisive effect on the ward staff. One staff nurse said of her post-registration experience of team nursing, for instance:

> It probably wasn't a good example because they didn't have a sister at the time and the D grades seemed to be running riot ... Sometimes it was like the ward was totally split down the middle; it didn't matter if you were on your knees on one side of the ward, the rest just sat there and gave advice.

Alternatively, team nursing was not favoured by many because it seemed inappropriate for Smith Ward. The charge nurse reiterated a number of colleagues' views when he said that team nursing would be difficult to introduce because of organisational constraints. It was seen necessary to move patients around the ward to cope with new admissions if male and female patients were to be kept in separate bays and if post-operative patients were to be easily observed. Although sceptical about 'climbing on band wagons', the charge nurse stated that he had nothing against the concept of team nursing itself and would welcome some of its implications, such as the greater opportunities it would allow him to give patient care.

Despite collective reservations about the mode, team nursing was introduced onto Smith Ward towards the end of the research project in response to external pressures, most notably the need to implement the named nurse system. Nurses on the ward thought that team nursing would allow them to meet this standard of the Patient's Charter through identifying the leader of a patient's team as their 'named nurse'. The way in which the named nurse initiative – and the subsequent need to reorganise nurses' work – was imposed 'from above' was resented. Nonetheless, some nurses thought the change to team nursing would bring positive advantages, such as rotation of the co-ordinator's job, which would help develop the skills of E and F grade staff.

PERCEPTIONS OF PATIENT ALLOCATION

The nurse is assigned a case load of patients for the duration of her/his span of duty. Nurses are responsible for carrying out the nursing care for that case load, with assistance for those elements of care outside their ability. The principle of this system is to give total care to a group of patients for a designated period of time. Whilst this attempts to individualise care, continuity is sacrificed to the shift system.

(Royal College of Nursing 1992a)

Patient allocation tended to be unpopular among nurses on Jones Ward, again because of the lack of continuity of care that they associated with the organisational mode. In this system, nurses were seen to be 'shunted about' according to the idiosyncrasies of the staff rota:

> You didn't get to know any of your patients because you went in one day and you looked after certain patients and you went in the next and it was totally different – the other side of the ward or something. There was no continuation of what you were doing. (Associate nurse)

Nurses felt that they had little control in other ways, too. Decision-making took place in a hierarchical way, and nurses seemed to feel that information might be actively withheld by more senior staff. For example:

> The thing that used to get me about [patient allocation] wards was this person being in charge and running about with this diary, and this diary was kept secret! All the facts of the whole ward were in this diary, and it just didn't make sense to me that no-one else knew what was going on except this person; it just seemed like organised chaos really. (Associate nurse)

On Smith Ward, however, most nurses were convinced that patient allocation was the most appropriate organisational mode for their particular situation, especially as they felt it offered them a way of 'opting in' when it came to offering continuity of care. As one senior staff nurse said:

> We do get good continuity with [patient allocation], but people have the option if they don't want the continuity – which is quite nice because we do have some difficult patients, so people don't have to stick with them all the time.

To summarise, the majority of nurses on both wards felt that the organisational mode they used was the most appropriate for their current situation. This appropriateness was judged in part according to the kinds of practical constraint that existed locally, such as the nature of the patient group (for example all male patients or a mix of both sexes), the geographical layout of the ward and the staffing levels. Thus in terms of practical considerations, there were clear differences between the wards, which helped to account for their different organisational approaches; a broadly similar commitment to patient care on both wards had been differently shaped by local constraints.

However, whether or not an organisational mode was viewed favourably also depended on how the process of nursing itself was constructed. In this respect, clear ideological differences began to emerge between the nurses on the two wards. On Jones Ward, for example, primary nursing was valued because it was seen to allow a greater continuity of care and, subsequently, a greater rapport and depth of knowledge concerning the patient. At the same time, primary nursing appeared to endorse nurses' sense of themselves as independent practitioners, made evident, for example, in the direct links that existed between the nurse providing care for an individual patient and members of the multidisciplinary team. On Smith Ward , continuity of care was not valued in the same way and patient allocation was viewed positively, partly because it allowed both continuity and discontinuity of care. Such flexibility was clearly linked to the nature of the ward's work and case mix. The potential to change the allocation of patients was desirable in order that 'heavy' work and 'dirty' work (frequent lifting and cleaning after incontinence) could be shared out among staff. It was also thought that staff should have the possibility of moving on if they found relationships with patients were becoming overly difficult or demanding. Yet the possibility of individual discontinuity also tied in with the way in which the ward's entire nursing staff were perceived as a team rather than individual practitioners; individual nurses were seen as equal, almost transposable units, despite the recognition of different skills, personality and experience. For nurses on Smith Ward, both primary nursing and team nursing were seen to work against this collective approach.

One of the clearest points to emerge from discussions with nurses about organisational modes was that it cannot be assumed that the introduction of primary nursing, by itself, is evidence of a more progressive approach to nursing, or suggests a greater commitment to patient care than exists where other ways of working are employed. A similar commitment to care may be differently expressed, according to local conditions, the priorities that shape the organisation of care, and the impact of either one of these upon the other. With this point very much in mind, the next chapter looks more closely at nurses' perceptions of care.

6

Emotional and Physical
Aspects of Care

INTRODUCTION

Care has been seen as 'the essence and the central, unifying and dominant domain to characterise nursing' (Leininger 1988, p.3). Yet, as a concept, caring is elusive, complex and open to a range of interpretations (Bartle 1991, Brykczyńska 1992), to the extent that its meaning remains unclear (Swanson 1991).

Although caring is still a loosely defined concept (Dunlop 1986, Chipman 1991), many theorists recognise a distinction between caring *about* someone and caring *for* someone. In general, to care about someone suggests an attachment or an emotional relationship but implies little about carrying out practical activities or devoting time to that person. In contrast, caring for someone implies providing for that person's needs without necessarily suggesting anything about affection or affinity (Ungerson 1983).

In the sociological literature, this distinction between 'caring about' and 'caring for' has often been associated with a (false) dichotomy between informal and formal spheres of care; 'caring about' is identified with unpaid care, emotion and the private domain, while 'caring for' is linked with paid work and the public domain. Because of these associations, care within the domestic domain is assumed to be superior (Ungerson 1990), even though caring relationships in the public sphere are often characterised by love and affection (Qureshi 1990) and the domestic sphere can be the site of violence and degradation (Barrett and McIntosh 1982). As Thomas (1993, p.663) has argued, the balance between work and emotion in relationships of care needs more attention, particularly as:

> The whole issue of emotion is dealt with in a rather confusing and one-sided way in much of the caring literature. It is confusing principally because no clear

50

distinction is made between: i) the privately experienced emotional or feeling state of the person doing caring work; ii) the publicly expressed 'emotional input' of the carer in the caring relationship (Hochschild's [1983] concept of emotional labour is clearly of relevance here), and, iii) the privately experienced emotional or feeling state of the recipient.[1]

In the light of this debate it is significant that, within discussions about the 'new nursing', the meaning of nursing care appears to be shifting from the requirement of nurses to understand and address the patient's needs (caring for), towards a broader interpretation which includes both 'caring for' and 'caring about'.[2] Research that looks at the meaning of care in nursing practice supports this view. Swanson's (1991) research, for instance, based on the views of patients and clients, confirmed her theory of caring, which includes the process of being 'emotionally present'. This means 'more than understanding another's plight; it is becoming emotionally open to the other's reality' (p.163). She notes that although there may be a sharing of feelings, what distinguishes this form of caring from others is that the nurse cares without obliging the patient to follow suit: there is no expectation of reciprocity.

According to Chipman's research among American second-year diploma students, behaviours considered to be 'caring' included 'meeting patients' needs in a timely fashion', 'providing comfort measures for patients and their families' and, significantly, 'giving of self'. According to Ersser (1991), such giving of self may be made evident in the way in which the nurse presents herself to the patient, and this 'presence' may have a bearing on the patient's well-being. In a preliminary account of his study of patients' and nurses' views on the therapeutic and anti-therapeutic effects of nursing, Ersser (1991, p.80) finds that:

> both nurse and patient participants continue to consider the effects of the nurse's presentation and presence on the patient at least, if not more, important than their specific-procedural actions.

This shift of emphasis which characterises the 'new nursing' – the importance given to making public what was previously the private, subjective sphere of the patient (and perhaps the nurse) – has been commented on by May (1992), who believes that it raises interesting issues of power and control. He suggests that in encouraging patients to reveal their innermost fears and emotions, nurses risk disturbing the balance of power in the nurse–patient relationship, which has previously been weighted in their favour. While the patient, in the face of disease or illness, has little choice but to comply with the demands of health workers regarding 'objective', clinical matters, he cannot be compelled to submit to demands regarding his subjective world (May 1992, p.599):

While the power to define and respond to the patient as more than the object of clinical attention rests with the nurse, it should not necessarily be assumed that practices through which subjectification is undertaken render the patient powerless. In fact, the opposite may be true.

Hockey makes a rather different point about power or control. She draws attention to the way in which, in contemporary Western culture, the concept of 'care' is rooted in a Christian concept of love and coexists in uneasy proximity with a concept of 'control', grounded in a scientific view of the natural world (Hockey 1990, p.183):

> Remaining always in tension with one another, control, as a limiting, dehumanising practice, readily evokes the cultural requirements for care – and care, a form of love which brooks no discriminations or constraints, rapidly brings exposure to 'problems' and the cultural requirement that they be controlled.

Hockey notes that just as religious beliefs and practices are regarded as matters of *individual* choice, so too is 'care' offered in the form of *individual* acts of humour, generosity or ingenuity.

Such issues of power and control contribute to the controversy that exists both inside and outside nursing regarding the role of caring in professional relationships (Swanson 1991) and raise a number of important questions regarding research into 'care'. For example, is caring a process that is observable in the behaviour of the care-giver or can it only be identified by the recipient of care? Rather differently, if research into caring is only now beginning to address the way in which, historically, cure has been valued above care (Chipman 1991) – if we have a scientific tradition that is 'blind to the very existence of the phenomena under study' (Graham 1983) – have the appropriate methods been developed to research this phenomenon?

This research did not attempt to elicit in any detail the views of patients regarding care. This was simply not possible within the time scale of the study. Instead, the study concentrated on the explanations that nurses offered regarding their interpretation of 'care' as well as the actions observed that might be construed as caring behaviour. Admittedly, such behaviours have been defined as 'caring' in a rather *post hoc* manner. For example, while some forms of touch have long been recognised to convey care, humour and posture generally have not been viewed in this light. While I was interested in humour prior to fieldwork because I thought it would help to indicate the nature of social relationships in the field, it was only after hearing nurses' comments about humour and examining the data from participant observation that I began to think of humour as a *means* of offering care, rather as Hockey (1990) had done. A similar developmental process applies to my perspective on posture, although I had not really anticipated that this would become a focus of the research prior to data collection.

Later in the book, specific nursing actions which appeared to represent or indicate care will be discussed. This chapter will be concerned with understanding certain dimensions of care, as seen through the eyes of nurses and made explicit in semi-structured interviews. Beyond the concept of 'care' itself, we discussed associated notions of 'love', 'closeness' and 'intimacy', mainly on my instigation; these notions have received varying degrees of attention in the nursing literature but all seem to lie somewhere near the heart of theoretical approaches to 'care'.

The numerous references to 'closeness' in the context of a therapeutic nurse–patient relationship have already been discussed in Chapter 2. Intimacy has been described by Meutzel (1988) in terms that are reminiscent of 'closeness', indicating that intimacy between a nurse and patient makes partnership in care a more concrete reality. Nurses are recognised to have the opportunity to develop emotional 'closeness' through the provision of intimate physical care (Ersser 1991). In addition, the work of Lawler has been important in highlighting the 'highly complex considerations' that are revealed in any attempt to understand how nurses deal with the physical intimacy they have with patients. Lawler (1991, p.29) draws a clear link between expert nurses' care of the patient's body and a more general category of caring, which is evident through the ways in which nurses manage physical care and their intimacy with the patient:

> Nurses ... help people with the experience of living with and through what is happening to their bodies during illness, recovery or dying – times when the body can dominate existence. Nurses are therefore centrally concerned with the object body (an objective and material thing) and the lived body (the body as it is experienced by living people). They are concerned with integrating the objective body with the lived body.

Thus, Lawler suggests that encouraging the integration of the lived body and the object body can be understood as a central element of nurses' care. Yet, it would also seem that this form of care, in which nurses employ their knowledge of the patient's experience of the body during 'basic' nursing activities such as bathing or giving injections, represents an example of how nurses simultaneously 'care for' and 'care about' the patient.

Besides recent recognition of the centrality of physical *and* emotional intimacy to 'care', increased emphasis on the affective dimension of nursing is sometimes expressed as a suggestion that nurses *love* their patients as part of their caring role. Jourard (1964), for instance, hopes that nurses will realise that nursing is 'a special case of loving'. Wright (1990) has described nursing as 'a healing presence with patients and [nurses'] involvement with patients takes a form of love'. According to Wright (1990, p.35):

> This love requires respect for the individual on the part of the nurse, a genuine desire to help another human being in what might, at the very least, be difficult and distressing times.

Campbell (1984, p.35) suggests that there is a tension in caring between a 'doing to' and a 'being with', and, in this context, nursing possibly offers a form of love that is a 'skilled companionship'.

The interest in this study was to see to what extent these notions of 'care', 'love', 'closeness' and 'intimacy' were central to everyday practice for nurses, and whether they had particular meaning for those nurses who, through the adoption of primary nursing, have rightly or wrongly become more closely identified with the 'new nursing'. Beyond this, if these notions came to shape nurses' practice, they might have implications for the support that nurses might need.

THE NOTION OF CARE

The ways in which nurses on the two wards perceived the notion of care were broadly similar. With the exception of one nurse on Jones Ward who described care essentially in terms of carrying out the nursing process or *prescribed* care, all nurses on each ward spoke of care as a response to the physical *and* psychological or spiritual needs of the patient. One staff nurse from Smith Ward, for example, explained 'care' as:

> fulfilling all [patients'] needs, whether they be physical or psychological. Where they've got a deficit, where they're not able to do something, we do it for them ... assist them where they would normally be independent ... It's not just physical care, it's caring for the whole. You know, if they've got psychological needs that overtake their physical needs, then that's what you would see yourself going on more.

In addition to this core understanding of care, nurses suggested other dimensions of care, which appeared to be expressed slightly differently by nurses on the two wards. On Jones Ward, a number of nurses referred to the importance of empathy and, often less explicitly, of being non-judgemental and understanding the patients' needs as elements of caring. For example:

> I think [care is] a combination of things ... you have to be interested in people to start off with, because if you're not, then you just come and do whatever it is you have to do for them and that's it ... I think it's an attitude as well ... whether [you] respect people as individuals – I think that has a lot to do with caring. And whether [you are] non-judgemental ... you can't always have empathy with everybody, but trying to be aware of what it's like for the patients, I think that's important. (Senior nurse)

Alternatively, on Smith Ward, nurses made less reference to empathy and instead stressed the centrality of talking to patients – of developing good rapport and communication – to the giving of good care:

When I think that I've looked after a patient well, I think half of it was establishing a good rapport between yourself and the patient so that the patient opens up, so that perhaps you get to something behind the physical problems as well. (Senior staff nurse)

This comment is reminiscent of May's (1992) reference to a new emphasis on revealing the subjective world of the patient, which he believes poses new issues of power in the nurse–patient relationship. However, as the following comments of the charge nurse indicate, rapport can be built on conversation in which the private world of the patient or nurse is not explicitly revealed, that is where there is no 'opening up'. Not only this; he also expresses an uneasiness about the 'right to know everything' about a patient:

Well, there is a case for serious conversation, obviously, and that's very important, but I'm also talking about very ordinary sort of commonday conversation that you would have with anybody ... It doesn't always have to be deep, psychological, sort of so-called counselling going on   you're just getting to know them. I think sometimes we just presume we've got the right to know everything about patients when ... it's up to them to really share what they want to share with us. And sometimes, there are things that are really difficult to talk about and ... I'd rather know that person a bit more first. So, I mean sort of social, ordinary interaction, like 'How are you today?', 'What did you do this morning?', 'Are your relatives coming in today?', you know.

Despite being more closely identified with the 'new nursing', nurses on Jones Ward gave no more stress during interviews to conversation with patients than did nurses on Smith Ward. Although, unlike nurses on Smith Ward, they were able to spend a good deal of their time sitting and talking with patients, 'talking' was not explicitly referred to by many nurses in their elaboration of the concept of 'care'. As stated earlier, the importance of offering 'empathy' or a non-judgemental understanding of patients' needs was stressed instead. This understanding need not necessarily be put into words but might be expressed in a more tacit way. A short case history from Jones Ward demonstrates this kind of approach, in which verbal interaction is not necessarily privileged. It also gives some indication of the nurse's implicit view of care, in the context of her relationships with other health workers.

A CASE HISTORY

This case history relates to the relationship between one of the primary nurses, 'Jane', and an elderly patient, 'Lee', whom she had nursed over a period of approximately three years.

As far as Jane could remember, Lee had been told that he had cholangiocarcinoma before they first met; as Jane put it 'He always seemed to know' and would refer to his diagnosis quite openly. Following the insertion of a metal stent to relieve an obstruction to drainage of the bile system, he had remained fairly asymptomatic for quite some time. Occasionally, the stent would become blocked or infected. When this occurred, he would contact the unit to arrange readmission and arrive shortly afterwards by taxi, always unaccompanied by his family. Typically, he would start antibiotic treatment, undergo endoscopic retrograde cholangio-pancreatography (ERCP), have his stent unblocked and go home, again by taxi. He was very independent. In terms of nursing, he required little in the way of physical care, and, as Jane put it, 'We spent more time talking than anything else'. The conversation was mostly about his life, such as his childhood in China, and his family. There were relatively few discussions about his illness or diagnosis. According to Jane:

> because he'd been in so many times for the same procedure he knew why he was coming; he knew what the matter was, and he knew what the outcome would be, so you didn't have to spend time reinforcing that. So really it was just conversation. He'd ask quite a lot about you, what you did. One afternoon he spent quite a lot of time teaching us to write Chinese, explaining the characters and things. He spoke a lot about his family. It was often the same sort of thing, but it was never boring or repetitive . . . He was never sad until his last admission.

On this last occasion, Lee was obviously quite unwell. For the first time, he was vomiting and feeling cold. According to Jane, he said, 'This is different. This admission is different to the others'. Jane relayed this perception to the house officer because she felt it significant, particularly as the house officer had never met Lee before. However, treatment started on the basis that this was a straightforward blockage of the stent.

Lee became weaker and weaker, and Jane saw that he was beginning to realise that, this time, he would not recover:

> I'd go over to him to do anything – talk to him or sort a drip out – and he'd burst into tears; for no particular reason it seemed – I just caused him to cry. It didn't seem a bad thing; it seemed to be quite nice, because if someone can cry in your presence, it says quite a lot. In fact, he didn't do it with anyone else . . . He said that whenever he saw me he just wanted to cry . . . I'd just sit and hold his hand, for ages really. We didn't particularly talk about anything; I can't remember what I said.

Eventually Lee was referred for an ultrasound scan, which showed multiple abscesses of the liver. Lee was told in the ultrasound department that there was little more that could be done for him. According to Jane:

> When he returned to the ward the pharmacist was just by his bed and he said to her, 'Oh, they've told me they can't do any more'; he was quite matter of fact about it. And then the pharmacist said later that she'd been struck by the fact

that when I came over to him, he'd instantly burst into tears and told me the same thing. She moved away quite tactfully, and I pulled the curtain round and spent quite a lot of time with him. But she told me later that she realised then what a difference in relationship there was between her and him and myself and him.

Members of the medical team expressed the opinion that Lee was denying the reality of the situation, a view very different from Jane's:

I said to the doctors that I felt he had accepted it . . . he might be denying it a little bit . . . it's only natural to want to keep on living; it doesn't mean to say that you've not accepted [the inevitable]. So he did used to talk to me about dying; he said he didn't want to die but he said, 'I'm old, my body's old and I can't live like this'. There was obviously a real battle going on – he didn't want to die but there was no alternative really.

By this time Lee was very weak, but he remained as independent as possible, usually staggering out to the bathroom to wash himself. He spent most of his time in bed, cocooned in his Chinese jacket, often asleep. Nurses provided pressure area care and offered small acts of comfort, but the majority of his care was still in terms of interaction. He would still talk about his family and ask about Jane's life outside work, but as he became still weaker this changed:

it was more just sitting on his bed. And he'd give you a look and just shake his head – it was a lot like that. Or he'd say, 'Oh Jane' and reach out and hold your hand. He became quite sad when he wasn't crying. Then he'd swing into being quite happy.

Reflecting on their relationship after his death, Jane said:

I think you can always underestimate how important you are – without blowing your own trumpet. I suppose it made me realise how much importance [patients] do attach to a person, or two or three people they've known for quite a long time. And the fact that you can communicate without . . . that you can cut the formalities really . . . *that you can communicate at a different level* . . . It made me ask a lot of questions about the way you look after somebody; you can't just write it in the care plan as something you should do. (my emphasis)

It was my impression that this 'communication at a different level' took place on both wards. Nevertheless, on Smith Ward, nurses did not generally have the opportunity to spend time with patients, so the empathic act of 'sitting with patients' featured less in their accounts. A further difference stemmed from the religious views of some nurses on Smith Ward; one of the senior staff nurses, for example, was a nun who was frequently called upon by other staff to see a patient if it became clear that he was anxious or troubled. Thus, there were one or two nurses on Smith Ward who 'specialised' in a form of verbal communication in which existential matters were explicitly discussed. This may have been because they had a pre-existing form of discourse, independent of nursing, which provided a basis for this approach, yet even these nurses expressed their lack of confidence about working with patients who were terminally ill.

LOVE

Nurses' views on the role of love within the provision of care suggested some subtle differences between the two wards. All the nurses interviewed indicated the complex nature of the word 'love' and suggested that there were different forms of love. Nonetheless, contrary to the views on love expressed in the 'new nursing' literature (see Wright 1990 for example), nurses on Jones Ward were almost entirely of the opinion that 'love' was either an inappropriate term to describe the emotional content of relationships between nurses and patients, or that it was an inappropriate emotion for nurses to feel for their patients. Love was generally an emotion reserved for a partner, 'family' or close friends, and, while patients were often regarded *as if* they were family or friends, there was (with very rare exceptions) a clear difference. One primary nurse expressed this in the following way:

> I would only use the word 'love' in relation to my family or to some of my friends, but then, when I think about some of the patients that I have nursed, they do become more like friends because you nurse them so much … although I've never seen any patient outside the hospital context, so there is that sort of barrier to it. I don't feel I can use the word 'love' in relation to a patient; I'm not comfortable with that.

A number of nurses were concerned that if the nurse–patient relationship was based on some form of 'love', nurses would be less well placed to offer appropriate care and support; they would be seen as too *close* to nurse effectively. 'Loving' patients suggested that nurses were too involved. It was important for nurses to maintain a certain distance from patients and to have some boundary to their emotions. Thus, by implication, nurses practising the 'new nursing' based on 'close' relationships would seem to have to strike a fine balance between developing 'closeness' and maintaining 'distance'. This suggests that nurses develop skills in 'placing' themselves in relation to the patient, both physically and emotionally, a point that will be discussed further in Chapter 7 and developed in terms of the implications for nurses' support needs in Chapter 9.

Three nurses on Jones Ward were sympathetic to the idea that nursing incorporated an element of love, although it was a moderated form, a love 'in your own sort of way'. One nurse thought that 'love' might be used to refer to the intensity of pleasure attached to working with certain patients. However, most nurses on this ward were more comfortable using the term 'care' rather than 'love'.

On Smith Ward, however, nurses were more prepared to use the term 'love' to describe their involvement with patients. It was thought that now nurses were encouraged to get to know their patients more and to treat them as individuals, they became more attached to patients, and that this attachment could be referred to as love. It was, however, only one form of love and quite distinct from the love that an individual nurse might have for a spouse or parent.

There was an additional way of understanding love, articulated by the charge nurse in the following way:

> Well, you know what the Jesuits say about love. They say love is not an emotion, it is an act of will. So when you're talking about love ... do you mean an emotional feeling towards [patients] – a good feeling, like tenderness or compassion? Well, I don't necessarily call that love. I mean, I would call that just being caring, because you don't like to see another human being suffer. I think my idea of love now would be when you have some patient who is, frankly, very difficult; you don't particularly like them and you find it very difficult to look after them. You don't get on, they're demanding – whatever – and you still go through that care-giving, and you do it to the optimum and the best of your ability. To me, that's love – when the going gets rough, you're still hanging in there. It's not an airy-fairy kind of good feeling.

One of the senior staff nurses, the religious sister, said in a similar vein:

> It's probably easier to love somebody than it is to like somebody ... Yes, I do think you should 'love' your patients (in inverted commas) as much as possible, because I think for a patient to begin to feel better, perhaps [they need] to feel accepted, feel they're wanted where they are and to feel that people understand them – and I think that all these things come under the umbrella of love.

She saw that not liking the patient made this more difficult but that dislike was ultimately irrelevant for the professional carer.

One of the other staff nurses, a born-again Christian, stated that she did love patients and suggested that this allowed her to be firm or directive when this was in the patients' interests. For example:

> I've got a relationship with them in that I can ... not tell them off, but say to them, 'Stand up, you're not holding your weight!' They know that I love them, that I care for them, that I make them comfortable; they don't have a horrible nurse.

This same nurse then went on to remark on how she had learnt to love patients to a large extent through the example offered by other, senior staff on the ward:

> I must admit I've learnt that on here though. I mean *some* of that's in me; I suppose it has to be a point in your character. But [it's also] role model. The senior staff nurses here, they're very loving and caring – you know, affectionate, have a laugh with patients, treat them as human beings.

In summing up, she distinguished the love she had for patients from that she might have for family and friends, seeing it as:

> a love as in 'I'll do to you what I want done to myself'. You can't always do it but . . . you're at least striving for that.

Thus, in very broad terms, a distinction appeared between the two wards. In one, nurses tended to describe their involvement with patients in terms of 'caring' for them, an involvement that might exceptionally develop into a closer kind of attachment, which was similar to, but still distinct from, the love experienced for family or friends. On the other ward, a number of nurses thought that love might almost be a precondition for care, particularly in the case of 'difficult' patients. This form of love, however, was not exactly a spontaneous emotion but more an act of will, a principle. On this ward, love was, at least for some nurses, implicit in the notion of caring, rather than one end of a continuum of emotions that might arise through giving care.

What was particularly interesting was that different perceptions of love (either as a precursor or an element of care) bore little relationship to nurses' stance regarding the 'new nursing'. Nurses on Jones Ward who identified more closely with a nursing-as-therapy approach did not uphold the views of 'new nursing' theorists such as Wright (1990), at least those views that concerned love. Alternatively, nurses on Smith Ward, who tended to be rather sceptical about the 'new nursing', appeared more open to using the term 'love' when referring to care, although they probably used the term in a different sense from those protagonists of the 'new nursing' who have advocated the importance of love. These rather surprising findings serve to remind us that nursing ideology may not be accepted in its entirety when put into practice, or may be cross-cut by other beliefs. In this instance, it is possible to glimpse the influence of nurses' sociocultural background – on Smith Ward, for example, the impact of some of the more senior nurses' religious beliefs – in shaping ward staff's understanding of care as a theoretical construct.

CLOSENESS

There were no clear differences between the wards in terms of the way in which nurses perceived 'closeness'. This was rather surprising, given that primary nursing has become associated with recognising the importance of the development of 'close' relationships between nurses and patients. Instead, views were heterogeneous within each ward. There was just one exception to this; on Jones Ward, two nurses saw closeness in terms of partnership, while none of the nurses on Smith Ward referred to it in this way.

Very often, closeness implied that the nurse knew the patient very well and that nurse and patient felt at ease with each other. In this sense, closeness was described as a kind of rapport. Closeness might also suggest a mutual acceptance, referring, for example, to a relationship in which it was possible to talk about anything without embarrassment or to say anything, however unwelcome or challenging this might be. This appeared rather similar to what Meutzel (1988, p.111) has described as 'a joint unmasking' in the therapeutic relationship. In this sense, closeness marked a largely unconditional relationship. Some nurses took a similar view but saw the nurse–patient relationship as less reciprocal: patients might be free to say anything to their nurse but nurses were more circumspect or less 'open'.

A number of nurses considered that most relationships would become close if there was sufficient contact over time. Others felt that only a few relationships would ever become close. Whether or not this happened would depend on at least one of the parties to the relationship 'opening up' about their feelings and anxieties; closeness occurred only when a degree of trust had developed. One or two nurses referred to the way in which closeness developed from the general interaction nurses had with patients. One senior staff nurse on Smith Ward said, for instance:

> you have a close relationship with most patients because of the intimate things you do for them, or help them to do, or talk about. You know, just saying to someone, 'Have you had your bowels open today?' – I think you need to have quite a close relationship.

Alternatively, she suggested, nurses may be the only people patients will talk to about trauma or grief, partly 'because you are the one they are closest to in the hospital environment'. This conflation of physical and emotional closeness is a constant feature of the data, a point we shall return to later.

Other nurses described an apparently similar view in which a distinction between closeness and attachment was more explicit; these nurses saw that it was necessary to be close to a patient in order to give care properly, but that one might not be attached to all patients or get on equally well, despite being close. This seems to correspond with the view that it is possible to love patients without liking them. In other words, the terms 'love' and 'closeness', as employed by nurses, need not *necessarily* imply affection but rather suggest a sense of understanding, which is personally less costly for the nurse to sustain. This possibility is important in understanding the support needs of nurses.

There was a very small group of nurses who felt that they only rarely, if ever, established close relationships with patients. For example, the charge nurse on Smith Ward said:

> I can remember one or two [patients or relatives] where they told you all about the ups and downs of their marriage, and why they didn't have children, or what

she was going to do with the flat after he'd died and, you know, all those kinds of things. I could have told them a lot of things about myself that I wouldn't necessarily tell anybody, that's closeness. Sharing something – that I might be fed up on a particular morning or something may have happened at home, and I'd be able to say, 'Well, actually this has happened and I'm just fed up' . . . I can think of only about half a dozen [patients or relatives] in the last few years, so that's my idea of closeness.

On Jones Ward, one nurse felt that she did not establish close relationships with patients. For her, closeness was more than empathy. It was about feeling what the other person was feeling, but, significantly, it was to be found only with friends and family. In fact, she was aware that while some patients related to the ward staff as 'family' and perceived the ward as 'home', she felt that this constituted an unhealthy dependence on the ward staff.

Other nurses' perceptions of closeness, however, included getting to know patients to the extent that it was possible to anticipate at least some of their needs or for the nurse to share the patient's experience to a certain extent. For example:

I think it's being part of it with them really. I think it's a certain intimacy that you get; every step that they go through, with their problems and their illness, you go through it with them . . . not necessarily experiencing it but being so close to them that everything that happens to them you want to know about, to care about it . . . it's to do with sharing what sort of things they are going through, really. (Senior nurse)

Similarly, one of the staff nurses on Smith Ward felt that closeness was about putting yourself in the patient's position, saying, 'I've always thought, "What if that were me sitting there – how would I feel?"' Alternatively, it was described in terms of being 'as one', suggesting that 'closeness' might be understood in some instances as being close to the 'same' (as discussed in Chapter 2). In this sense, nurses' use of the term 'closeness' seems to offer a glimpse of a broader understanding of certain categories, such as 'personhood'. For example, some nurses' use of the expression 'closeness' suggested a view of the person as not always clearly bounded and divisible, a perspective that is not generally represented in nursing models but may, nonetheless, underlie aspects of nursing practice. (The concept of individuality will be returned to in Chapter 7.)

What was also notable was the way in which nurses used physical terms to describe social relationships with patients. Chapter 7 argues that nurses' use of metaphors such as 'closeness' reveals an implicit assumption of mind–body unity – an assumption with important implications for nursing practice. For now, attention will merely be drawn to the way in which nurses might talk about 'being with' or 'opening up', or, classically, about their 'closeness' to a patient in ways that suggest a conflation of the physical and the non-physical. For example, one nurse said she would explain 'closeness' as:

> well, I suppose in terms of physical closeness, and then there's closeness that comes from knowing somebody . . . so when I say 'closeness', I mean both really.

As a participant observer, I was struck by the way in which physical proximity, for example during a distressing procedure, seemed in itself to represent 'closeness' – that physical closeness could both signify *and* foster emotional closeness. This overlap between the physical and metaphysical is perhaps not surprising among nurses; what they experience and learn in the course of their work runs counter to a mind–body dualism. Moreover, it raises interesting questions about the meaning of intimacy between nurses and patients.

INTIMACY

The conflation of physical and emotional closeness that underscores many nurses' accounts also occurs when they discuss what it means to give physically intimate care in the context of an emotionally close relationship. As with 'closeness', there is no trend that characterises either ward team but rather a range of differing views within each. Overall, the majority of nurses found it easier to carry out intimate procedures, such as giving suppositories, with patients they felt 'close' to. For example:

> The closer I feel to a patient, if I have to do something that's particularly intimate or particularly unpleasant, then I find it much easier because I can say to them, 'Look, this is really awful and I'm sorry if it's embarrassing for you' and they say, if we are close and they know me, 'Well, it's OK, it's you, I know you', sort of thing. (Senior nurse)

Many of those interviewed also thought that carrying out intimate procedures might help in the development of close relationships.[3] As the health-care assistant on Jones Ward said:

> I think the majority of people, where I've had to be intimate with them, you know, I think it's helped . . . It's broken the ice . . . There's many a time when I've said, 'Come on, how about getting you in the bath . . . you'll feel better and I'll wash your hair for you' . . . Yes, it helps a lot I think.

Although these comments are initially surprising, they can, on reflection, be seen to support Lawler's (1991) argument that nurses focus on the integration of the lived body and the object body. However, there were certain circumstances in which the same group of nurses became uneasy about intimacy. One such situation was where the age of the patient was similar to that of the nurse, particularly (but by no means exclusively) if the patient was of the opposite sex. The patient's personality and how he coped with the process of being a patient was also relevant. Moreover, if the patient was exceptionally 'close' – for example, a very good friend who became a patient – this could lead to profound embarrassment and avoidance of any intimate contact. For example, one primary nurse said:

> If you're as physically intimate with a close friend as you are with a patient . . .
> I mean, you would ask a colleague to go in and do it because it would be embar-
> rassing. It doesn't *necessarily* mean that the closer you are to somebody, the more
> physically intimate you can be with them.

This corresponds with Lawler's (1991) findings. Some nurses in her study found it difficult to nurse people they knew, some found it made little difference and others found it highly satisfying. The nature of the experience, however, seemed to depend upon the patient, the nature of the patient's condition and the kind of pre-existing relationship. Significantly, Lawler (1991, p.161) found that having an established *social* relationship generally interfered with the development of whatever is specific to the nurse–patient relationship:

> It is impossible to summarise easily what transpires between a nurse and a
> patient, because it is such a complex social phenomenon, and it varies with each
> individual encounter. What is clear . . . is that the social climate of the
> nurse–patient relationship is a special kind of relationship.

Pre-existing acquaintanceship or friendship tended to restrict the development of a relationship conducive to professional conduct and the performance of care.

The study data indicate, as the discussion of 'love' suggested earlier, that for many nurses, there was a clear demarcation between emotions appropriate to the ward and the emotions reserved for 'outside'. The following chapters will help to show that non-sexual physical intimacy was possible within the ward, largely because of the symbolic meanings attached to this clearly bounded world; the nature of the ward as a *symbolic* space allowed specific and non-sexual interpretations of nurse–patient intimacy. Before elaborating on this point, however, it is worth noting from the example of friends-as-patients how relationships originating outside the symbolic space of the ward appeared to have the effect of weakening the particular 'reality' that was constructed within it.

Significantly, the 'closeness' that the majority of nurses referred to was similarly defined and circumscribed by the context of the ward: a 'close' relationship was one that might be *modelled* on relationships that occurred outside the hospital but, nonetheless, differed from such relationships.[4] This was also made clear by the importance that nurses attributed to uniform in allowing them to carry out intimate procedures. It appeared that uniform helped nurses to manage intimacy with patients by transforming nurses into representations rather than specific individuals. One primary nurse said, for example:

> you put on your uniform as a nurse and that gives you access to, you know, things that you just wouldn't do to . . . it's outrageous really but a nurse's uniform, a nurse's title, status, gives you . . . like a passport to do all these things. It's incredible really.

It was interesting that nurses on Jones Ward had carried out research concerning nurses' uniform, with a view to dispensing with it altogether. After a few months, however, nurses became convinced, contrary to their expectations, that uniform played a useful role. As one primary nurse noted:

> I remember when we did the non-uniform experiment, and I had a young chap, same age as me I guess, and I had to do some intimate things and he was acutely embarrassed because I had my own clothes on, so I was a person, not a nurse in his eyes. And I found that embarrassing because I knew he was embarrassed.

What this example suggests is that, in order to facilitate the giving and receiving of care, nurses and patients collectively construct a particular kind of reality (see Berger and Luckman 1967). This will be expanded on in Chapter 8, where it will be suggested, for example, that on Jones Ward, the nature of the nurse–patient relationship is made clear by the construction of a context that is more domestic than institutional in character. In this chapter, however, we have glimpsed how, if the context in which this relationship is located is transformed too completely from an institutional to a private sphere, the definition of reality that nurses and patients abide by becomes unhelpfully ambiguous. Thus, we can see that the construction of reality that informs nurse–patient interaction is not only complex, but also highly fragile.

SUMMARY

In this chapter, we have again seen how organisational mode and nursing doctrine are mediated by other factors, such as local conditions. For example, nurses on Jones Ward could offer patients care in the form of 'presence' because of adequate numbers of staff. A number of nurses on Smith Ward saw 'loving the patient' as integral to care due to their religious beliefs. 'Closeness', meanwhile – recognised as one of the central features of primary nursing – is equally important to nurses on both wards, perhaps because it is a cultural construct that plays a central part in structuring many relationships both inside and outside nursing.

In addition, we are beginning to see evidence, through notions such as 'closeness' or the way in which nurses view intimacy with patients, of a fusion of bodily and psychological domains. This phenomenological understanding of nurse–patient interaction and its role in the provision of care is further examined in Chapter 7. It will suggest that nurses' use of touch, their choice of metaphors and the forms of humour they employ represent tangible expressions of nurses' embodied knowledge.

ENDNOTES

1. See also the work of James (for example 1989).
2. This study addresses to some extent the issue of whether or not an institutional context, such as that of a hospital ward, can be seen simply as a public domain; that is, it comments on the dichotomy that is drawn between public and private spheres of care.
3. There were two nurses whose views seemed to represent exceptions to this trend. One, a nurse from Jones Ward, said of giving suppositories, 'The more I know a patient, the more I feel that I'm intruding'. The other nurse, from Smith Ward, said, 'I feel more conscious of an invasion of privacy when it's someone close'. What is interesting about these comments, apart from their similarity of content, is that they were made by nurses who were unusual in stating that they very rarely formed close relationships with patients; they tended to reserve this term for social or family relationships.
4. A point that has significance for those nurses working in local communities where it is difficult to draw a distinction between, on the one hand, the symbolic world that defines the meaning of the nurse–patient relationship and, on the other, the 'outside' world and the social relationships that occur there. I am grateful to nurses who attended the St Mary's Past and Present League address (Savage 1993), who observed that nurses who worked in small communities, and thus knew many of their patients socially, would perhaps construct a context for care that was very different from that of Jones Ward.

7

Interaction and Nurses' Embodied Knowledge

It is now widely recognised that nursing knowledge is complex and varied in nature. Carper (1978) has identified four different patterns of knowing in nursing:

- empirics (the science of nursing);
- aesthetics (the art of nursing, including intuition);
- personal knowledge (self-awareness and reflection);
- ethics (moral knowledge).

While nursing involves all these diverse forms of knowledge, these ways of knowing have historically been given different emphasis or value. Traditionally, nursing has been shaped by empirical knowledge (or logical empiricism), but today there is also some readiness to accept other 'patterns of knowing' less amenable to scientific scrutiny. Nursing is increasingly seen as 'a particular kind of interpersonal interaction' (Clark 1991: p.376), about developing and sustaining relationships with people (Kitson 1987, p.328), but with expert nurses unable to articulate all that they know (Benner 1984).

It is important for the development of the discipline of nursing to find ways of exploring nurses' 'ways of knowing' (Vaughan 1992). Yet expert knowledge, because it is largely tacit in nature and, thus, difficult to describe, presents researchers with methodological problems (Kitson 1987, MacGuire 1991, Meerabeau 1992).

This chapter looks at nurses' interaction with patients, with a view to eliciting the unspoken knowledge that underlies it. The interaction in question may be verbal or non-verbal but suggests a form of knowing that appears not to fit Carper's taxonomy. Instead, it simultaneously involves intuition and experience. This will be referred to as 'embodied knowledge', to emphasise its non-intellectual nature and, at the same time, to draw attention to the way in which it suggests and/or reinforces a unity of mind and body, the physical and the existential. This suggestion (if not promotion) of unity fits with Kitson's (1987, p.323) premise that nursing 'must involve seeking that which maintains unity between body and soul'.

Previously, the term 'embodied knowledge' has been used in at least two ways in connection with nursing. Benner and Wrubel (1989) suggest that nurses' embodied knowledge enables them to act in rapid and non-reflective ways, particularly in activities where the physical and the cognitive are intertwined and where, indeed, conscious thought may disrupt the execution of complex skills. In contrast, Lawler (1991), as we saw earlier, suggests that nurses have a knowledge of the body (somology) that is associated with 'integrating the object body with the lived body' (p.29). It is an understanding, on the part of the nurse, of the patient's embodiment. As used here, however, 'embodied knowledge' also refers to an integration of the *nurse's* object body and lived body, in relation to others. This aspect of embodied knowledge will become clearer in Chapter 8. The current chapter represents an initial exploration of nurses' tacit knowledge of the patient's world. It approaches this knowledge through looking at how nurses make use of touch, humour and metaphor in ways that apparently reinforce a psychophysical unity.

It has been recognised that language forms, such as metaphor, as well as gesture and other actions, may hold symbolic meanings, which may be associated with healing (Kirmayer 1993). The main purpose of this chapter, however, is not to attempt to reveal the therapeutic process that may be initiated by a 'close' nurse–patient relationship; that would be far beyond the scope of the study. Instead, it is hoped to show how nurses' use of forms of communication (such as touch or forms of rhetoric) helps to reveal the embodied knowledge on which much of their practice rests.

TOUCH

Touch is recognised as central to care-giving and the nurse–patient relationship (Estabrooks and Morse 1992, Weiss 1992), with touch routinely involved in many nursing tasks. According to Lorensen (1983, p.179), touch represents:

> one of the nurse's primary tools for establishing rapport with patients within a short period of time and in meeting patients' needs.

Various typologies exist, but, beyond the very specific category of therapeutic touch, different forms of 'everyday' touch have generally been grouped under one of two main categories: *expressive touch* (sometimes called caring or comforting touch) and *instrumental touch* (alternatively referred to as task-oriented or procedural).

While there is a growing body of knowledge regarding nurses' use of touch (see for example Weiss's 1988 review), Weiss (1992) notes a general assumption that different types of touch carry the same meanings, leading to a focus on the *amount* of touch used rather than its qualitative dimensions. In a study of the reported use of touch by medical-surgical nurses, Farrah (1971) found that informants thought that touch has the capacity to convey positive meanings, such as support, the willingness to be involved and '*closeness*'. Similarly, Estabrooks and Morse (1992) observed that nurses often take it for granted that higher amounts of touch have positive implications for patients. However, for patients, touch may be experienced as a way in which nurses exercise control (Mulaik et al 1991). In her review article, Weiss (1988) also comments that the meaning of touch may not always be a positive one for patients, and notes that it is not clear whether touch increases or decreases patients' anxiety. A number of studies that she reviews suggest that the interpretation of touch will depend on the specific relationship between a nurse and patient, as well as on a range of variables such as age, culture or the part of the body touched. Similarly, Morse (1983) finds that the appropriateness of touch is linked to the degree of trust and intimacy that exists in a relationship. Thus (Weiss 1988, p.5):

> Rather than having universal meaning, the meaning of touch gestures may be context-dependent and person-specific.

This research did not set out to study touch, yet it was found during field-work, particularly on Jones Ward, that nurses' use of expressive touch was so remarkable that it became an important focus of the study. For example, on Jones Ward, during the bedside handover, nurses made continuous efforts to involve patients by using touch at strategic moments. It was also common at other times to see nurses holding hands with patients while they sat and talked. I also experienced this heightened use of touch, both through finding myself touched by staff from my earliest visits to the ward and through realising that, after spending some weeks on the ward, I used touch with patients to a far greater extent than ever before. On Smith Ward, the use of touch was less obvious, at least between nurses and patients. This is not to suggest that nurses used expressive touch less than nurses on Jones Ward, but that nurses on the two wards used slightly different forms of expressive touch, which will be described in more detail later.

On both wards, nurses frequently used touch with their peers, whether this was to offer comfort, keep a colleague's attention or express solidarity. Touch was also involved in the horseplay nurses indulged in, either as an element of a joke or as reassurance, a way of countering the meaning of the joke. For example, when one off-duty student nurse came to Smith Ward to enquire about the shifts she was to work, she was clearly interrupting the nurse in charge, who pretended to kick her on their way to the ward office, as if taking revenge. Once at the door, this ostensibly aggressive behaviour was qualified when the more senior nurse gently stroked the student's back.

Such observations led me to raise the subject of touch during interviews. In these, nurses indicated that non-instrumental touch had a range of effects. This expressive form of touch was seen, for example, to make links between a nurse and a patient, to offer reassurance and to convey understanding of distress. Thus, for some nurses, touch became a representation of care. Others, however, emphasised the therapeutic potential of touch; it could be 'uplifting' or enable patients to 'open up'. Touch could help patients to relax or (important for later discussion) to 'feel at home'.

The use of touch was also reassuring for some nurses; nurses felt more confident in their interaction with patients when their use of touch was accepted by patients or when patients touched them (see Adair 1992 on this point). Touch was seen to indicate a degree of 'closeness' between the nurse and patient, and a recognition of that closeness.

Significantly, while some nurses explained their positive attitude towards touch as a result of their own family attitudes, a few nurses also remarked on the way that they might readily use touch within their role as a nurse but not a great deal in their family or social relationships. Several nurses thought that they had become more tactile as a result of nursing. In addition, one or two nurses referred to the way in which general life experience (as opposed to nursing experience) had contributed to the way they used touch. For example, one nurse spoke of how she had received ultrasound as therapy for back pain and had found the use of a machine without any accompanying use of touch quite unsatisfactory:

> I remember feeling really not cared for; all I could feel was this machine. Now I'm more aware when I give IV drugs, take somebody's pulse or something – all sorts of little things we do – to have some contact as well. You see lots of people giving IV drugs and [they are] just sitting there watching the drug go in. I feel sure [patients] would like some human contact as well, so I just put my hand on the side of their hand or just stroke the vein above where the drug is going in.

This comment suggests that the distinction between instrumental and expressive touch may not always be clear. The reference to a *deliberate* use of non-instrumental touch points to the possibility of a range of different forms of touch within the overall category of expressive touch.

This suggestion is supported by the views of a number of nurses, particularly on Jones Ward, who thought that expressive touch was used in different ways according to the experience of the nurse. Junior nurses were seen to use touch more spontaneously, and nurses with more experience were thought to use it in a more considered way. One associate nurse spoke of how a very junior nurse had 'overdone it' by using touch in a way that she considered to be indiscriminate. As one of the primary nurses put it:

> I suppose if you're aware that there are different types of touch, then, as you became more senior, you could deploy them as you judged appropriate, whereas as a junior student you would just use touch in a spontaneous, natural sort of way, and this may be inappropriate.

Student nurses did, in fact, often describe their use of touch as spontaneous. For example:

> I mean, one of the patients was telling me how he lost his eye nastily at a party, and, I said, 'Oh no!' and touched his arm – you know, my arm just *went*. (Third-year student, Jones Ward)

Although I observed nurses using touch more frequently on Jones Ward, the senior nurse there expressed some doubt that an emphasis on touch was, as such, linked to the ethos of primary nursing. It was, however, associated with the closeness of the relationship between a nurse and patient. This might mean, she suggested, that because the continuity of care made possible by primary nursing allowed the potential for closer relationships, touch was used more often by those employing primary nursing.

However, although I was more aware of the use of touch on Jones Ward during participant observation, a number of nurses on this ward said in interviews that they did not use touch a great deal in their work; they might express this as being 'not very tactile'. These nurses, nonetheless, were observed using non-instrumental touch – particularly during handovers. Here (as mentioned in Chapter 3), it seemed that touch was rarely used in a way that was entirely spontaneous. Instead, a conscious attempt was made to use touch as a method of 'involving' the patient in the handover. For example, one primary nurse said:

> We say when we do bedside handovers that we should have contact with the patient so that they feel involved ... I'm sure that as patient, I would feel isolated and cut off to hear people talking about me close by ... I'm sure I would automatically feel involved if I was included [by touch].

Interestingly, this nurse thought that the ward standard concerning handovers stated that touch should be incorporated, although what it actually required was that the nurse conducting the handover should sit close to the patient. Moreover, this recommendation was included primarily for reasons of confidentiality rather than any explicit recognition of the importance of involvement or inclusion for the patient.

Nurses' use of touch was remarkable during handovers not only because of its frequency, but also because it was surprisingly uniform in kind. Touch was used in more or less predictable ways, suggesting that it was not spontaneous, nor necessarily dependent on the patient's circumstances. This way of using touch was not viewed favourably by all nurses. One associate nurse on Jones Ward who, it should be noted, often took an alternative stance to others on the ward and, for example, felt that she did not develop close relationships with patients, observed that touch lost its value if used all the time. One staff nurse from Smith Ward, who had worked once or twice as an agency nurse on Jones Ward, made a similar observation about non-verbal communication in general:

> I've noticed it there and I've just felt it was very false, their communication. You know, they go up to [patients] and get down to the same level ... they've read that in a book; they know they've got to do it. I didn't think it was flowing naturally.

Here, as in an earlier quote, the term 'natural' appears to imply spontaneity, and it is in the varying attitudes towards spontaneity that differences concerning expressive touch emerge between the two wards; among the permanent staff, touch appeared to be used in a more considered way on Jones Ward.[1] Initially, during participant observation, expressive touch appeared to be used less on Smith Ward, but in fact what was absent was the *formalised* use of expressive touch. This was borne out by interviews with Smith Ward staff, in which only spontaneous expressive touch was referred to. A striking example of this form of touch was given by the charge nurse:

> We had one particular man who was very distressed one day, and we had a student nurse – standing next to me – and [the patient] said something to me and ... I just kind of stroked his cheeks [as if to say], you know, 'Poor fellow'. And this nurse next to me started crying! I said, 'What's wrong with you?' and she said, 'Oh that was so beautiful!'. I said, 'What? ... What have I done?' I thought I'd done something wrong! She said, 'The way you touched that person' – and I wasn't conscious of it.

To some extent these differences in the use of touch may be influenced by the different styles of nursing found on the two wards, but the distinction between the two wards is not entirely clear cut. The same charge nurse, for instance, also described how he might give some of his elderly female patients a peck on the cheek. This was not a spontaneous gesture but a conscious acknowledgement of their maternal feelings towards him, made explicit, for example, in the way they referred to him as 'a lovely boy'. Indeed, the influence of the ward ethos regarding touch was cross-cut by a number of factors, such as the age of the patient, their social class, the sex of the nurse in relation to the sex of the patient and their respective personalities.

The sex of the nurse seemed, in itself, to play little part in the readiness to use touch, as the charge nurse's statement above demonstrates. Most nurses, both male and female, commented on how rarely they used touch with young men (that is men of a similar age to themselves) because of the risk that this might acquire a sexual connotation. However, this reluctance was generally overcome where the patient was in distress or in contexts where there could be no misinterpretation of the nurse's action.

Significantly, a student nurse training predominantly at a children's hospital found it easier to use touch with children, largely because there was little risk of it being misinterpreted. I was able to observe her work with an agitated, adult patient attributed with a mental age of two years and found that the use of touch, especially in the form of hugs, formed a major component of her care. Her almost total body contact with the patient, made possible by the asexual status he was ascribed, was clearly successful in calming him and was acknowledged by other nurses and patients to represent a high quality of care.[2]

Unlike the considered use of touch during bedside handovers on Jones Ward, the spontaneous use of touch was not articulated or promoted by either ward in any concrete way. At the same time, although a considerable number of nurses said that they used touch spontaneously, at least on some occasions, there was a general agreement among nurses on both wards that nurses were, nonetheless, often selective in the way in which they used this form of touch. However, decisions about when or how to use touch were not made in a conscious manner. Many nurses were at a loss to describe quite how they made these decisions. Others said that they just 'knew' from experience what was appropriate in a particular situation with a particular patient. Many nurses referred to the 'vibes' that they experienced from patients, which informed them whether or not touch would be acceptable. Some nurses thought that their decisions were at least partly informed by the patient's body language, for example by whether or not they crossed their arms, although the assessment of body language was not something that the nurse was aware of doing. Having said that, it is entirely possible that the patient's expectations regarding touch – and thus his body language regarding his receptiveness to touch – were influenced to some degree by the general ethos of the ward and what he saw going on around him.

There was some agreement among nurses that the 'intuitive' knowledge they had regarding when and how to use touch was not entirely the result of their experience as a nurse. Some degree of this knowledge was thought to be present before training, as a type of general social skill, but it was then developed or heightened through nursing practice. This concurs with the observations of Estabrooks and Morse (1992), who describe the process of learning touch for a new intensive care nurse as follows (p.452):

She begins to listen, to observe role models and to place herself 'in the patient's shoes'. She rapidly identifies nurses whom she wishes to emulate and learns intensively from them. This learning includes how these nurses interact with patients and how they touch them. Although informants explained this process, they could not recall ever explicitly thinking 'That nurse is touching in a way that I will try'. Rather, it was the total behaviour of the ideal nurse, of which touch was a part, that they sought to adopt.

Nurses' use of touch and the way in which nurses shape the context in which touch occurs appear to have something very important to say about the nature of a non-theoretical knowledge that nurses develop, a point that will be returned to later. Before this, we shall see how the same sort of knowledge becomes evident through nurses' use of humour.

HUMOUR

Humour has been studied by social scientists as a way of understanding social relations (Radcliffe-Brown 1940, Coser 1959, Douglas 1975, Mulkay 1988, Fox 1990, Hockey 1990, Dwyer 1991). For example, in hierarchical organisations, humour tends to reinforce the existing structure (Coser 1960, Mulkay 1988). Where hierarchy is less formal, humour such as reciprocal joking may help to express and even enforce equality (Howe and Sherzer 1986). Among a number of studies that look specifically at humour within organisational life, Coser (1959, 1960) has found that humour among hospital staff often signifies the rejection of a rigid authority structure, although it might also be used by those in authority to mask the power that they hold. Dwyer (1991), in addition to seeing humour as the product of power relations and a way of contesting those relations, suggests that intragroup humour can be a tool for the construction and defence of group identity.

It has also been noted that the relationships marked by joking are often characterised by a combination of friendliness and antagonism and tend to occur in situations where, for some reason, there is ambiguity. Significantly, the world of nursing is full of ambiguity. In the provision of physical care, context and intent are all that differentiate some nursing actions from sexual ones (Savage 1987). According to Littlewood (1991, p.170), nurses become equivocal figures through dealing with 'the disruption of normative time and space caused by sickness', and the management of ambiguity becomes a central task of caring. Furthermore, nurses appear to use humour in the management of this ambiguity. Hockey (1990) has observed, for instance, that nurses' work in residential homes for old people often brings them into contact with processes of disease, ageing and dying, where there is no clear boundary between life and death. Both nurses and residents appear to use humour to cope with these indistinct categories.

Beyond this inherent ambiguity, nurses may also *create* moments of indeterminacy through their use of humour. In a sociological analysis of humour, Mulkay (1988, p.4) has suggested that:

People employing humour temporarily inhabit not a single, coherent world but one in which whatever is done and said necessarily has more than one meaning.

Because of its ambiguity, humour can sometimes be used to introduce topics that nurses or patients otherwise find difficult to broach (Emerson 1973). Because humorous statements need not be taken seriously (according to Mulkay [1988, p.217] 'humour becomes directly subordinated to the demands of the serious domain'), a joke can be used to negotiate the introduction of an otherwise taboo subject, yet still be dismissed as 'only a joke' if the initiative is not favourably received. Similarly, Hockey (1990) has suggested that some things become known through practice and *only* reach the level of discourse through humour and allusion.

This approach to humour is useful, as it suggests that the study of this phenomenon in nursing may help to identify those situations in which a plurality of meanings either pre-exists or is intentionally created; understanding nurses' use of humour may help to show how nurses cope with or even manipulate ambiguity. In this way, it may tell us more about the nature and use of nurses' non-theoretical knowledge.

Humour has also been seen as an integral part of recovery and as a means of providing a sense of caring, although there is little understanding of the circumstances under which humour becomes a therapeutic intervention (Sumners 1990). Theories concerning the possible psychological and physiological functions of humour are outlined by Robinson (1977) and Ruxton (1988). Howe and Sherzer (1986) describe how, in many societies, having to laugh at one's own misfortune or hearing others do so becomes an obligatory way of coming to terms with adversity, which protects the unfortunate from the strong emotions of gloom, resentment and anger. Lawler (1991) finds that nurses often use humour as a technique to help themselves and their patients manage difficult situations by minimising the size, severity or significance of a problem. Similarly, Ruxton (1988) suggests that humour can neutralise emotionally charged events. As we saw earlier, it may encourage people to risk messages that, if regarded as serious, might be unacceptable, and so offers a way of initiating communication on taboo topics (Emerson 1973).

Despite this recognition of the use and value of humour, there is little information regarding its use in the practice setting and little exploration of what humour means either for nurses or patients (Simon 1988, Sumners 1990). One way in which humour appears to be of relevance to this particular study is touched on by Robinson (1977), who suggests that, besides having the potential to relieve anxiety, convey emotional messages and reduce muscular tension, humour (like touch) also helps to establish *rapport*. As we have seen earlier, nurses in this present study have seen 'rapport' as either a component of or a synonym for 'closeness'. Humour may, therefore, play an important role in the development of a therapeutic nurse–patient relationship.

The issue of how and why nurses use humour was of interest prior to the fieldwork, as a result of anecdotal evidence that suggested there was less humour where primary nursing was practised. This apparent change in the use of humour might, for example, suggest a change in the distribution of power between nurses and patients. Had this interest not predated field-work, humour would, nonetheless, have become a focus of the research as, during data collection, it became clear that humorous exchanges were an important element of nurses' relationships on both wards. Nonetheless, nurses' humour at work was a most difficult subject to study; as Fox (1990, p.443) has noted, 'writing an ethnographic account of humour is like trying to put Humpty Dumpty back together again'. As humour was not recorded *verbatim* (except where it was used during interviews), only some very general observations arising from the fieldwork and a report of what nurses themselves had to say about their use of humour can be given here.

Nurses' perceptions of humour

On the whole, nurses on both wards understood the effects of humour in similar ways. Nurses' use of metaphor in describing these effects is striking. For example, humour was seen to *break down barriers* between patients, or patients and staff, or to *break the ice*, suggesting that humour could be used to bring about change within social relationships.

Alternatively, humour was 'therapeutic' in that it could *lighten* the atmosphere by *lifting* patients or cheering them *up*, and helping them to forget their problems for a while. The following comment by a senior nurse on Jones Ward suggests that, in *lifting* patients' mood, humour has a therapeutic potential:

> I mean, to think about patients on this ward particularly . . . they all have fairly miserable diagnoses – dreadful chronic conditions . . . a lot of them really suffer . . . I do definitely think it's therapeutic; to have people that are fairly prepared to lighten the day a little bit [by joking with them] makes a big difference.

She went on to explain that humour's therapeutic potential lay in the way in which it could bring about a more positive mental state, which, in turn, might lead to a better outcome.

One of the most striking ways in which humour's therapeutic effect was described both by permanent staff and students was in terms of relieving stress or *relaxing* patients. As one senior staff nurse said regarding the use of humour:

> When you're a patient, as I've been myself, you're a lot more vulnerable, so I think whatever can make you feel less vulnerable, more relaxed, *more at home* is going to contribute to making you feel a little bit more yourself – and to improve your sense of care and improve your sense of well-being as well. I mean, for patients within hospital, I think a sense of vulnerability is far . . . far deeper than I think we can really actually appreciate . . . things have to be done to create a

sense of safety for the patient, and to work from there in the sense of making them feel more at home in order to let them relax more and, hence, improve their recovery. (my emphasis)

This statement is particularly interesting in the way it links relaxation through humour to being 'at home'. There is an association between well-being and being 'more yourself' which is, in turn, associated with the private sphere or home; the home or the family are widely understood in Western culture as the location of the *real* self (Cannell 1990). The significance of 'being at home' was a recurrent theme in the data and is discussed later. However, it is worth noting at this point that, as in the case of touch, the use of humour may help to produce a particular kind of social reality, and transform a hospital setting into a quasi-domestic setting.

Humour was also important in relieving stress among nurses and, here too, its effect was described in metaphorical terms. For example, one nurse referred to the way in which humour helped to 'keep your head above water'. It also *lightened* the nurses' situation. A primary nurse on Jones Ward, for example, said:

I think humour is a large part of your work really in your relationship with colleagues. I think if you're in a stressful environment, it's a stop-gap; you can avoid *blowing a fuse* by having a laugh, by *lightening* things, and it acts as a support mechanism. I think most of the staff have a good sense of humour, which does help; people are very supportive, and I think humour's got quite a bit to do with it.

Similarly, a senior staff nurse on Smith Ward remarked on the importance of humour for raising staff morale, saying, 'it just *lightens* the atmosphere, which can sometimes be quite *heavy*'. She went on to give an example of a situation in which humour had been used supportively, something that had occurred that very day during the afternoon handover:

They had a cardiac arrest this morning and the patient [pause] didn't make it, and then the patient in the bed next to him is also terminal – and you could sense almost when the nurse [gave the report] . . . you can imagine how she was feeling after the morning. I'm not quite sure if it was [the charge nurse] threw in some kind of joke (you know, 'Come to Lourdes' kind of thing, 'and all will be made well'), and it just kind of *lightened* the atmosphere really.

As in the case of touch, virtually all nurses referred to the importance of using humour appropriately, but, again, precisely how nurses knew what was appropriate was difficult to articulate. Although it was agreed that much depended on the patient and the nurse's knowledge of the patient, there was no consensus on either ward regarding how the knowledge represented by the nurses' use of humour might be conceptualised. Indeed, several nurses expressed two, apparently opposing, views within the same interview, suggesting that (as with touch) knowing how to use humour is based on both 'spontaneity' *and* practice. For example, one staff nurse said that knowing how to use humour 'just comes naturally. The most important thing is to listen . . . You have to know when it's appropriate'. However, when asked how she knew when it was appropriate she replied:

> I don't think I do really. I don't think you know until you've said it, and then you know it wasn't really appropriate. I don't think it comes naturally; I don't know actually, it might do but it certainly comes with practice and being around people; you get to know how people are and how they will react. Well, I don't think about it actually . . . I'm more likely to think, 'Oh I mustn't do that here' rather than 'I must do that here'. (Staff nurse, Smith Ward).

Observations of nurses' use of humour

Humour often took the form of mild bantering or mock rudeness. In this, the impressions from the study are similar to those of Hockey (1990). She found that, in the residential home, humorous exchanges often represented attempts on the part of nurses and patients to play with the forms that constituted their situation and their relationships. Hockey (1990, p.179) says of rudeness between staff and patients:

> [by] being rude to each other, they have asserted the sense of closeness and intimacy which they have developed in the course of their extended relationship.

On the two wards in this study, the use of rudeness was apparent between staff and patients with long-term relationships, but it was also observed among nurses and 'new' patients, suggesting that this form of humour might also be used as a way of building or even accelerating the development of relationships towards intimacy or 'closeness'.

The relationship between power and the use of humour was not explored in any depth. As stated earlier, Coser (1959, 1960) has suggested that humour among hospital staff often signifies the rejection of a rigid authority structure, although it could also be used to conceal power. I found some possible support for both of these seemingly contradictory arguments. At least one, relatively senior, nurse stated that she used humour to get round awkward situations with more junior staff on the ward. This apart, nurses often made themselves and their colleagues the butt of jokes with patients, encouraging patients to treat them with apparent rudeness. Dwyer (1991) has noted that the literature on humour suggests that 'marginally placed actors' often use joking as a strategy to make themselves more central, by entering into a coalition with the joke's audience at the expense of its target. Given the emphasis on partnership and patient empowerment associated with the 'new nursing', it is interesting that nurses in this study tended to make jokes at their own expense. This use of humour might represent an attempt not so much to mask but to redistribute the power that nurses held in their relationships. Significantly, several nurses commented that they liked it when patients began to tease them, interpreting this as a positive comment on the patient's morale and on the nurse–patient relationship.

Paradoxically, humour was widely recognised among the nurses spoken to as a means of allowing their personality to become evident – to 'counter the effects of the uniform'. Yet, it seemed to me that although the content of jokes could be improvised, the way in which humour was used conformed to certain patterns. For instance, jokes made with patients were often ironic in nature, with a disjuncture between what was said and what was meant. One example of this form of humour was offered by the senior nurse on Jones Ward, who asked a very frail patient to look after the ward in her absence and keep an eye on the nurses. In this instance, what made the nurse's statement humorous was that, in reality, the patient was too frail to accomplish the most basic tasks without assistance, let alone take on the management of the ward. The patient's frailty was, therefore, given acknowledgement, but through the inversion of reality. Patients often joked with nurses about how they would 'keep an eye' on one or more of their colleagues, implying that, as patients, they had a deeper commitment to or understanding of the nurse's role than some nurses themselves. Yet, the nurses such patients referred to were those on whom they were most dependent. It was as if, through the very act of being rude about the nurses' capabilities, these patients were acknowledging their dependency and *affirming* their confidence in their particular nurse. As one nurse said, humour is helpful for 'describing a situation', but from observation it seemed to achieve this through the use of paradox or contradiction.

These types of joke help to show the 'multiple realities' of the social world that Mulkay (1988) believes is addressed more adequately by humour than serious discourse. In the first scenario, for example, the joke may acknowledge the patient's frail condition, but it may *at the same time* make reference to the fact that, despite his physical frailty, the patient remains sharp-witted and observant. In addition, the joke pivots on the recognition that, in reality, it *is* nurses who are in charge of the ward; this aspect of the joke is cross-cut by the desire of nurses on the ward to redistribute the power they hold and develop relationships of partnership with their patients. Thus, the joke has not one but a number of meanings, each more or less intended, each receiving different degrees of recognition and collectively making reference to a number of realities.

This ability to relate to a multiplicity of meanings is not restricted to nurses in their use of humour; it has been recognised as an attribute of humour in general. Presumably, there is an overlap between the humour an individual nurse uses on and off duty. However, an awareness of nurses' use of humour helps to develop a wider picture of the complex skills and knowledge they employ as practitioners. For example, in this study, humour appeared to be a far more central component of the interaction between nurses and patients than it was between doctors and patients, or between doctors and nurses. Moreover, the humour was not wildly idiosyncratic or entirely dependent on the particular nurse and patient. Rather, humour appeared more of a collective strategy and was used in a largely similar way among nurses on each ward. A similar point can be made regarding nurses' use of metaphor.

METAPHOR

Metaphor is one of a number of figures of speech (or tropes) in which a word or expression is apparently used in other than its literal sense (Hawkes 1972). Historically, there have been two distinct linguistic approaches to metaphor, which reflect divergent opinion about the relationship between language and the world. According to one view, the *constructivist* position, metaphor is an essential characteristic of the creativity of language. The other, *non-constructivist*, view of metaphor portrays it as a violation of linguistic rules, an inessential frill that contributes little to our understanding of 'reality' (Ortony 1979).

The discussion of metaphor here falls very much into the 'constructivist' camp, characterised, for example, by the work of Lakoff and Johnson (1980). They suggest that metaphor is pervasive in everyday life because human thought processes are largely metaphorical. These authors argue that because metaphor is central to our conceptual system, the kinds of metaphor we use help to structure not only what we think but also what we do. They give the example of the concept of 'argument' and the conceptual metaphor that 'argument is war', showing how this particular metaphor is reflected in our everyday language through a wide range of expressions. In arguments 'opponents' take 'positions', which are 'attacked' or 'defended'; arguments are 'lost' or 'won'. Moreover, this way of conceptualising 'argument' comes to inform the very way in which we argue and the actions we perform while we argue. To clarify their point, Lakoff and Johnson (1980, p.5) ask us to imagine a culture where arguments are not seen in terms of war:

> Imagine a culture where an argument is viewed as a dance, the participants are seen as performers, and the goal is to perform in a balanced and aesthetically pleasing way.

In such a culture, people would think about, talk about, experience and carry out arguments differently, because the metaphorical concept of argument is different.

If our experience of the world is linked to our choices of metaphor, the study of metaphor would seem an important way of rendering our experience of the world more accessible. According to Lakoff and Johnson (1980), metaphor allows us to understand one kind of experience in terms of another. Metaphor, then, may be particularly helpful where we wish to understand what is inchoate and difficult to articulate in a literal form; according to Fernandez (1986, p.6), 'metaphor is one of the few devices we have for leaping beyond the essential privacy of the experiential process'. Thus, nurses' use of metaphor in references to nurse–patient interaction, such as their use of the expression 'closeness', may help us to understand their experience of this interaction.

Yet, even within a constructivist account of metaphor, there are disagreements regarding the relationship between language, knowledge and perception which we need to touch on, particularly with regard to the extent to which metaphor should be given a literal interpretation. One view is to see that 'the essence of metaphor is understanding and experiencing one kind of thing in terms of another' (Lakoff and Johnson 1980, p.5). What the speaker says in a metaphorical statement differs from what he or she means, and if a metaphorical utterance is paraphrased in order to express the speaker's meaning in a literal form, some element of meaning may be lost (Searle 1979). Searle gives as an example the way in which the rich meanings underlying Disraeli's statement 'I have climbed to the top of the greasy pole' are not adequately conveyed once paraphrased as 'I have after great difficulty become Prime Minister'. The literal statement offers less insight into what it takes to achieve success in a political career. Thus, metaphors 'may often serve to plug . . . semantic gaps' (Searle 1979, p.97). This suggests that literal translation of metaphorical expressions noted during this study may not be fully satisfactory, as there will be a gap between the meaning of the metaphorical statement and that of its literal paraphrase. In this case, it is probably unrealistic to attempt to do more than draw attention to nurses' use of metaphor and the apparent coherency of these metaphors.

However, there is an alternative way of approaching metaphors, which may help to give greater insight into the meaning underlying those used collectively by nurses. In this approach, instead of seeing metaphor as a way of saying something about something else, it is treated as if it is a literal statement (Overing 1985). Put slightly differently, instead of assuming that metaphor shows 'the thisness of that', it can be regarded as demonstrating 'the thisness of *this*' (Jackson 1989, p.142). According to Jackson, if metaphor is viewed in this way, it can help to reveal the psychophysical unity of human experience. He provides an example of how metaphor indicates this unity through observing how we 'fall' or are 'thrown' when our everyday life is disrupted. For instance, 'falling in love' or 'falling ill' are experienced as a simultaneous disruption of mind and body (Jackson 1983, p.329):

> In this sense, uprightness of posture may be said to define a psychophysical relationship with the world, so that to lose this position, this 'standing', is

simultaneously a bodily and intellectual loss of balance, a disturbance at the very centre and ground of our Being. Metaphors of falling and disequilibrium disclose this integral connection of the psychic and the physical; they do not express a concept *in terms of* a bodily image.

This approach to metaphor suggests that it may be possible to increase our understanding of nurses' lived experience regarding their interaction with patients through looking at their use of metaphors, particularly those 'orientational metaphors' that refer to bodily activity and stance.

Orientational metaphors

Lakoff and Johnson (1980, p.56) have referred to many of the kinds of trope that this study found to be used by nurses as orientational metaphors, which are linked to the kinds of body we have and to the specific ways our bodies function:

> We have bodies and we stand erect. Almost every movement we make involves a motor programme that either changes our up–down orientation, maintains it, presupposes it, or just takes it into account in some way.

According to Lakoff and Johnson, this spatial experience influences the structure of the concepts by which we live. Thus, we find a whole range of 'up–down' metaphors, which indicate, for example, that health and life are associated with 'up' (the 'peak' of fitness, Lazarus 'rose' from the dead), while sickness and death are linked to 'down' (we 'fall' ill or 'drop' dead). According to Lakoff and Johnson, this complex of metaphors has a physical basis inasmuch as serious illness forces people, literally, to lie down. They suggest that most of our fundamental concepts are organised in terms of one or more orientational metaphors, each of which has an internal systematicity; the association of health with 'up' is part of a coherent system – there is no context in which 'he is sinking' implies that a man's health is improving. Beyond this internal systematicity is an overall external coherence, so that the association of health with 'up' is matched by other states of well-being, such as happiness, that are also associated with 'up'.

Significantly, there are many possible frameworks for spatial orientation, besides that of 'up–down'. Other spatial concepts referred to by Lakoff and Johnson, but given less attention, include those of 'in–out' and 'near–far'. These refer to our experience of ourselves as bounded entities, separate from others, and 'containers with insides and outsides' (Lakoff and Johnson 1980, p.58). Put another way, some metaphors might be seen to refer to our cultural experience of individuality. Yet from the examination of nurses' choice of metaphor, it appears that nurses do not necessarily experience individuality in terms of discreteness and closure; or, at any rate, they suggest through the use of metaphors, such as those of 'closeness' and 'openness', that the ideal nurse–patient relationship and the therapeutic process are based on nurses' attempts to mitigate or soften individuals' experience of separateness and enclosure. In order to develop this point in more detail, it is first necessary to consider further the notion of 'individuality'.

INDIVIDUALITY

There is a clear trend in nursing of emphasising that patients need to be understood as 'individuals'. This appears to mean two things simultaneously. The first meaning concerns the patient's 'individuality', the understanding that each patient is unique in terms of personality and experience. This sense of being individual is superimposed on the second meaning of the term, that all patients are individuals inasmuch as the category of 'patient' can be mapped onto the physical body and that all such bodies are discrete or discontinuous with any other body. Particularly in Western culture, this individual human organism largely corresponds to the social category of 'the person', the unit of social significance with legal rights and moral responsibilities (La Fontaine 1985).

The view of the individual as a natural unit remains the focus in most areas of biomedicine, although defining the individual in terms of the biological body poses a dilemma even within a biomedical framework. For example, biologists cannot define any single developmental transition at which a biological individual with a clear, unique identity emerges, as debates about research on embryos have highlighted; from a developmental embryologist's perspective, individuality is a continuous process extending, perhaps, across generations (Johnson 1989). Nor is there an absolute scientific distinction between the biological body and the world it inhabits. In the field of immunology, for instance, what is self and not self, and whether the body stops and starts at the level of the skin, is brought into question by immunologists' views of autoimmune disease; as Haraway (1989) puts it, individuality becomes a problem of defence and comes to be understood in terms of disassembly or reassembly. She adds that individuality depends on context and that (1989, p.20) 'you and I . . . might be individual for some purposes and not for others'.

This is particularly clear in the shifting status of individuality experienced by women. As Haraway notes, women's bounded individuality is compromised by their reproductive role. The 'individual' that pregnant women carry within them during pregnancy may in some circumstances be granted greater recognition or precedence than themselves. Immune function during pregnancy also suggests an ambiguity regarding female individuality – generally, the mother's immune 'surveillance system' remains blind to the presence of the fetus (Haraway 1989). To summarise, the individual human organism, which is taken for granted within biomedicine as a natural entity, cannot be defined as a discrete unit except on the basis of social distinctions.

It, therefore, should not surprise us that, beyond biomedicine, what counts as 'the individual' is a matter of social rather than physiological definition. In some cultures, for instance, an individual is seen to be changeable in substance, although 'substance' in this instance is more metaphysical than physical. Where the caste system prevails, for example, 'individuals' have been characterised as malleable entities who can be essentially changed through the nature of their social exchanges and the ritual status of those with whom they interact (Marriott 1976). In Western culture, too, there is evidence to suggest that individuals are not necessarily perceived as divisible, bounded units but that their boundaries are dependent on conduct or context. In a study of English Catholics attending Lourdes, for example, Dahlberg (1987) describes how individuals are understood to be capable of physical, spiritual and mental change through contact with relics, holy places and objects. Finally on this point, it has been suggested that the view of the physical body as bounded is, anyway, one that only represents the experience of one, dominant group – that of heterosexual men – and does not necessarily reflect the lived experience of others within the same culture (see for example Code 1988, Savage 1992).

In this present study, nurses' use of metaphor suggests an understanding of the therapeutic process in which the person is neither isolated nor bounded, and that healing may occur where 'closeness' between nurses and patients is promoted by close physical and emotional proximity in the context of a (mutual) 'openness' or receptiveness. Thus, individuals, at least in the context of the 'new nursing', are ascribed the potential to change through proximity, contact, 'openness' and exchange with others.

In Chapter 6 we saw how nurses use terms such as 'closeness', 'being with' or 'opening up', which generally refer to physical relationships, to describe their social relationships with patients. Moreover, physical proximity – where, for example, the nurse might sit close to the patient and where there is, perhaps, some form of sustained bodily contact – might, in itself, indicate the existence of a psychic or emotional 'closeness'.

Like 'closeness', 'openness' has both physical and psychological dimensions. Several nurses referred to the way in which an 'open' stance was important in establishing 'closeness' or rapport; for example, it was felt that standing with arms crossed while talking with patients represented lack of 'openness' and a way for the nurse to maintain distance.

Of relevance here is Hockey's (1990) suggestion that the manipulation of social metaphors can profoundly alter experience and meaning in the case of ageing and death. She found that in both the residential home and the hospice where she worked, strategies of distancing and separation are part of these processes, particularly of dying. These strategies, she believes, are less obvious, but nonetheless pervasive, in the wider society beyond these specialised institutions. Here, in looking at how nurses understand healing, we find, instead of strategies of distancing and separation, those of bringing together or amalgamation (where the degree of 'closeness' brings about 'sameness'). We also find that nurses not only use metaphors to describe therapeutic interaction, but they also manipulate metaphors to bring about change in their interactions with patients, so, for example, sitting close both creates and affirms 'closeness'.

In this way, we can argue that, from a constructivist perspective in which metaphor is interpreted as if it has literal meaning, nurses' language, perception and knowledge have a certain coherency; if metaphors based on the body disclose the 'integral connection of the psychic and the physical' (Jackson 1983, p.329), it becomes possible to glimpse nurses' embodied knowledge or lived experience through their use of metaphors such as 'closeness'.

This 'articulation' of embodied knowledge through metaphor can be seen in other ways, too. We have seen how the use of humour was seen to 'lighten' and to 'lift', and how on Jones Ward, emphasis was placed on 'getting down to the patient's level'. Nurses felt it appropriate to sit or squat, that is to physically lower themselves in relation to patients, suggesting that patients, by virtue of being unwell and vulnerable, are in a different place from nurses but, nevertheless, one that nurses can attempt to gain access to. It appears that, through physically placing themselves in the patient's position of 'being down' – or as near as possible to this – nurses feel that they will comprehend what it means to be 'down' in a more existential sense. Taking the patient's position in a physical sense, in terms of being on a par, can also be seen as an initiative on the part of the nurse to create a greater degree of equality in the nurse–patient relationship.

Finally, nurses regularly referred to the way they approached patients in terms of 'going in'. This term often referred to going to see a patient whose bed was screened; 'going in' meant going in behind the screens. Occasionally, it referred to approaching the patient's space, as demarcated by the curtains, whether or not these were drawn around the bed at the time. In addition, there were other occasions when nurses would talk about entering the patient's emotional world in terms of 'going in' or 'going in there'. In this context, 'going in' appeared to refer to a potentially therapeutic moment when the patient might be 'open' to the nurse's intervention. This lack of clear distinction between the patient's physical space (the area of and around the bed) and other, metaphysical, regions is discussed more fully in Chapter 8, before looking more closely at ways in which nurses' use of the body may inform us of their lived experience, and of the relationship between the political space that nurses inhabit and the 'reality' that nurses create through their active use of the body.

ENDNOTES

1. This observation raises the question of to what extent nursing, or certain forms
   of nursing, can be understood as 'performance' and, if they can, what the implications of this might be. These points will be discussed in Chapter 8.
2. See Savage (1987) for a discussion of the growing emphasis in nursing literature
   on the assumed advantages of physical contact between nurses and patients.

8

'Closeness' and Symbolic Space

In this chapter, I shall be looking at how the hospital ward as a 'bounded' area can be viewed as a particular kind of symbolic space. This follows Hockey, who argues (1990, p 98) that, in terms of the residential home she studied, this particular institution:

> demonstrates the role of a boundary or frame in the creation of a time and space within which events or acts acquire expressive power, the meaning of which is open to interpretation.

While in the case of the residential home, separation between staff and residents is emphasised as preparation for the inevitability of death, data from the present study suggest that on the wards in question, the distance between nurses and patients is underplayed if not negated, both physically and symbolically. Nonetheless, the emphasis on 'closeness' varies between the two wards. On Smith Ward, a greater degree of separation is maintained, reflecting perhaps the particular case mix and/or the level of resources available. While, almost by definition, both wards *are* non-ordinary spaces, it becomes clear that, at least on Jones Ward, 'closeness' is not only stressed but also facilitated by a denial of the extraordinary context in which the nurse–patient relationship develops; nurses' actions serve to reclassify the ward as a domestic instead of an institutional space.

This 'reclassification' raises questions about the nature of these actions on the part of nurses, and the extent to which these can be understood as 'performance'. For example, what is the relationship between nurses' 'performance' during nurse–patient interaction and their 'embodied knowledge'? Before looking at whether or not it is helpful to think of nurses' actions in these terms, the issue of 'space' deserves exploration, as performance and space are profoundly interconnected. Thus, after a few words on the notion of privacy, nurses' explicit statements about space, and how they define this differently for themselves and their patients, will be presented. This is followed by an examination of how the space in which nurse–patient interaction takes place is differently constructed by nurses on the two wards, according to where they draw a boundary between the 'public' and the 'private'.

PRIVACY

Generally speaking, the term 'privacy' is taken to refer to the need of individuals, or perhaps families or other social groups, to *separate* themselves from others for certain activities or periods of time. In the Western world, privacy can be seen as a corollary of individualism; individuals are thought to have the 'right' to privacy (Sciama 1993). Yet (p. 87):

> the concept of privacy has no precise and uniform content; it is therefore very difficult to define, whether in ethical, psychological or simple linguistic terms.

What people may wish to keep private (for example affection, emotion, sexual activity, food consumption or the elimination of body products) may vary from one culture to another, and from one context to another. Thus, privacy can be seen as a continuum, with no fixed point at which the public becomes the private.

According to Lawler (1991, p.166), privacy has both concrete and abstract meanings for nurses:

> It can mean all of the following, either individually or in combination – a lack of audience, no unnecessary exposure of the body, minimising the possibility of embarrassment . . . maintaining a person's dignity, and an aspect of personhood.

She states that respect for privacy is a fundamental principle of nursing practice and informs many of the nurse's actions. In practical terms, for many of the nurses in Lawler's study (1991, p. 125), privacy meant:

> not over-exposing the patient, and it also means ensuring a visual privacy such that others cannot see the patient's nakedness. In effect it is dealing with the body in a privatised and 'civilised' way, but it is also somological – the nurse must 'do for' the body while simultaneously recognising personhood.[1]

According to Lawler, nurses in her study regarded embarrassment – for nurses and particularly for patients – as a consequence of inadequate protection of the patient's privacy. Yet it is beginning to emerge that 'privacy' is a complex concept. It appears to be dependent on perceptions of personhood and the extent to which people are thought to be separate (or, for that matter, 'close'), as well as on an understanding of what is public and what is private. Yet, as we have seen, these phenomena are rather nebulous or context dependent.

In the present study, nurses were not asked, as such, about how they understood privacy. Instead, they were asked to explain what they understood by the term 'personal space' in the hospital context. This area of questioning developed because of the way in which space was organised, particularly on Jones Ward, with remarkably little demarcation between patients' areas and nurses' areas. It seemed possible that there was a link between nurses' emphasis on 'closeness', a spatial metaphor, and the physical context in which nursing care occurred. This ties in with Sciama's view (1993, p.91) that, in studying the interaction of groups and individuals, the area of most interest is:

> the borderline between the private and the social and the ways in which privacy itself is patterned or organised in different societies. Thus states of mind, such as 'brooding', 'longing', 'grieving' or 'ecstasy', which in some societies are considered to be private experiences *par excellence*, are nonetheless culturally styled and delimited.

Using this approach, if we understand 'closeness' as a cultural phenomenon and a relatively private experience, which is conceptualised in spatial terms, we will perhaps learn more about it by looking at how 'private space' is understood and organised, and by observing the distinctions that nurses draw between their own personal space and that of patients (in other words, what is considered 'public' and 'private' from the nurse's perspective).

THE PATIENT'S PERSONAL SPACE

In the present study, nurses understood the term 'patient's space' in a number of ways. For example, some nurses gave the impression that particular areas of the ward 'belonged' to certain patients. When asked to describe the 'patient's space', the area defined was that taken up by the bed, chair and locker, plus the immediate area around the patient's bed. The boundary corresponded with where the curtains hung, whether or not these were pulled around the patient's bed.

Several nurses associated this sense of space with the notion of privacy, saying that the area around the patient's bed constituted *potential* 'space' for patients. It was not truly their 'space' as it was constantly invaded by a range of personnel, irrespective of the patient's wishes, suggesting that, ideally, patients' space referred to a physical or metaphorical domain in which patients had some control over whether they might be observed or approached.

As with Lawler's (1991) findings, the view that patient privacy was a fundamental need and right informed many of the nurses' actions. This was especially clear on Jones Ward, where, for example, nurses generally asked permission before going behind the curtains screening a patient's bed, often doing this by calling out, 'Knock, knock!', even striking the curtain with their fist on occasions, and waiting to be asked to enter. Similarly, the ward's Standard regarding the bedside handover placed a limit on the number of nurses who might enter the patient's space at any one time.

For many nurses on both wards, patients' 'space' simultaneously referred to the freedom that patients could exert, not only over their immediate surroundings, but also over their own person. Patients were seen to have 'space', for example, when their permission was actively sought prior to invasive procedures. Thus, personal space was not necessarily enhanced a great deal for those patients in cubicles or private rooms. Jones Ward had none of these, but some nurses thought that, in recompense, patients had more 'space' than on other wards, in that they had more freedom; if they were well enough, patients were encouraged to wander around the hospital or even the local shops. Similarly, efforts were made to free patients from unnecessary hospital routine, such as being woken at a set time in the morning. This freedom was often referred to by nurses as 'space'.

'Space' was also understood, particularly on Smith Ward, in terms of the patient's room to think. Patients were seen to have little space, not only in the sense that conditions were cramped, but also in that there were few opportunities for uninterrupted reflection; patients were badgered by a virtually continuous flow of nurses, medical students, domestic staff, pharmacists, doctors, visitors and porters. In this sense, the concept of 'space' overlapped with that of time.

THE NURSE'S PERSONAL SPACE

The perception of nurses' personal space was quite different. For example, there was apparently no temporal dimension to nurses' space; the term did not suggest 'space' for reflection, although it might refer to a sense of freedom or autonomy that they could experience in their work.

On Jones Ward, in particular, the concept of nurses' personal space was given remarkably little weight and, significantly, there was no space that was specifically demarcated for nurses. There was, for example, no central nurses' station, only a small desk on the ward for the telephone and relevant information, and nurses were actively discouraged from congregating around this. Administrative tasks and the writing up of nursing care plans were carried out at the bedside. In addition, there was an absence of any office or similar room specifically for the ward's nurses, although during breaks, staff could make use of a nearby room shared with nurses from a neighbouring ward. While there were strong links between the staff on these wards, a number of nurses stated a preference for some sort of private space on their own ward. There was a 'quiet room' attached to the ward – the place where most of the interviews with staff from Jones Ward were carried out for the study – but this was not routinely used by nurses. For the most part, this room was used to counsel anxious or distressed visitors, and although it was geographically linked to Jones Ward, it was also used by the adjacent ward for counselling purposes. Thus, there was no place for nurses periodically to escape the gaze or potential demands of patients or visitors, nor indeed a place where their identity as a team could be routinely reinforced.

For the majority of nurses, the lack of any private office did not pose a problem; some suggested that personal space was something that you carried around with you, rather than being a specific location. Only one or two nurses said that they found it difficult 'being on show' all the time, and this was particularly the case when they were not busy. Most nurses rapidly became accustomed to the lack of a nurses' station – often within a matter of days – and thought that the absence of a specific space for nurses fostered 'involvement' with patients. For example, one primary nurse expressed this clearly while comparing the arrangement on Jones Ward with other, more traditional wards:

> [There was always] our little corner or something – but no, I don't need that now. I don't know what I did, sitting there. I guess it was a bit of protection really, a sort of 'Oh don't talk to people for too long' . . . as they always say, 'Don't get involved with people – too stressful', but it's second nature now.

On Jones Ward, then, where there was a deliberate attempt to encourage interaction between nurses and patients and to minimise 'distance' between the two groups, there was very little distinction made between the nurses' space and that of the patients. More precisely, while nurses had little private geographical space into which they might withdraw from patients or others, and, indeed, were not seen to need private space, patients had little private space, although their need of such space was widely recognised.

Smith Ward was more traditional in terms of the way in which it organised nurses' space. There was a central nurses' station, around which nurses tended to gather, particularly towards the end of a shift. In addition, nurses used the charge nurse's office for tea breaks and for counselling or support from other ward staff. There was also a seminar room, which was used for teaching sessions and for the first part of the handover between shifts, besides being used by other hospital staff, such as the medical teams. These spaces, with the exception of the nurses' station, were quite separate from the patient areas and offered nurses a recess from being visually and audibly 'on show'.

Nurses on Smith Ward were, anyway, less visible than nurses on Jones Ward because of the different layouts of the wards. While nurses on Jones Ward were almost always on view to the entire range of patients on the ward, nurses on Smith Ward were for much of the time only visible to patients in a particular bay or cubicle. Ward layout therefore played an important role in determining the nature of nurses' space. Yet, beyond this, it was clear that nurses defined the boundary between themselves and their patients differently on the two wards.

This boundary however dissolved for nurses on both wards once they became involved in giving physical care. Nurses' close proximity with patients – for instance, while lifting patients – was something that they accepted without reservation; it was not experienced as an infringement of their personal space. Only in the case of sexual harassment, when their intimacy with patients was taken advantage of, did nurses notice a lack of personal space. Here again was an example of how, according to the views of nurses, the map of private and public space might be drawn differently for nurses and patients; patients required privacy and their bodies were private, although requiring the attention of nurses, while nurses did not require privacy (at least on Jones Ward) and their bodies were generally part of the 'public' domain while intimately involved in the giving of care.

Lawler has discussed how nurses use a number of strategies, such as the adoption of a certain manner, to recast situations so that the patient need not feel embarrassment; as she says (1991, p.154):

> Nurses must deliberately construct a context which allows the body and the embarrassment associated with exposure, dependance and illness to be managed in a particular occupational context.

Embarrassment, she suggests, occurs when social rules are broken, particularly those concerning 'privacy', and she implies that experienced nurses are able to redefine what is usually 'private' for the patient in order to minimise the embarrassment that nurses and patients are heir to.

Similarly, in this study, it seemed that nurses were able to manipulate the context in which nursing care took place, through redrawing the boundary between public and private, not only to alleviate embarrassment, but also in order to manage other aspects of their interaction with patients, including the development of 'closeness'. While this 'manipulation' is glimpsed in the way in which nurses define their own personal space in relation to that of patients, it can also be observed in the way that the symbolic space of the ward is shaped.

THE WARD AS A SYMBOLIC SPACE

Mention has already been made of the way in which a lack of rigid routine on Jones Ward was seen to give patients a degree of personal space. Yet, along with other measures that tended to downplay the institutional nature of the environment, it also helped to shape the ward as a particular kind of symbolic space in which events and actions were given meanings generally associated with the private rather than the public domain.

Benner and Wrubel (1989, p.394) have observed that:

Domesticating and thus normalising the highly technical hospital environments and the strangeness brought on by illness is a central coping resource for patients, families and nurses.

To illustrate their point, they give the example of an expert nurse who, when working on a coronary care unit, went about reassuring a newly arrived and anxious patient by saying, 'We eat cookies and laugh here, too'.

On Jones Ward in particular, the environment had been 'normalised' to the extent that, during participant observation, patients referred to the ward as 'a home from home' or commented that being readmitted was like 'coming home'. The only exception to this was the description by a patient who had spent all of his life in one kind of institution or another; for him the ward was 'wonderful! Like a hotel!'

Normalisation was not only brought about by the provision of domestic details, such as the use of a telephone for incoming calls or freely available coffee or tea. It also appeared to be achieved by the transposition of members of nursing staff into 'family' members. This was less evident on Smith Ward; although many nurses indicated that part of their nursing role was to make patients feel 'at home', the following discussion refers only to Jones Ward, where turning the 'extraordinary' into the 'ordinary' was more marked.

It has already been reported how, for staff, good care was generally understood as that which nurses gave *as if* caring for a family member or friend. Additionally, patients identified certain nurses as 'caring for me like a daughter' or 'like family'. As one primary nurse was told by the family of a patient whom she had known over several years, 'You're almost one of us'. This reclassification of nurses was evident in other ways, too. In terms of their public image, nurses have been widely and persistently portrayed as sexual objects; the common stereotype is of the nurse as the whore with a heart of gold (see Kalisch et al 1983, Salvage 1985). This public image can inform patients' behaviour towards nurses, who may experience verbal and non-verbal sexual harassment at work (Savage 1987, McMillan 1993). On Jones Ward, however, it appeared that nurses were seen in rather different terms. For example, one associate nurse said:

I remember one patient I had a few times, he made a comment one day. He was going on about nurses – the saucy image and things – and he said a really strange thing: 'We don't sort of view you lot on this ward as, say, *things*, like women walking down the street, sort of looking at their backsides. I suppose you're different because we respect you on the ward.'

From this, it could be argued that the female nurses on the ward were viewed not as women who were in the public domain (or outside the family), but as women in the domestic sphere who were not objectified in the same way.

Thus, through a number of means, the extraordinary situation of the patient (and, one might add, of the nurse) wrought by illness, hospitalisation and intimate care was apparently made more manageable by constructing an analogy between hospital life and family life. As suggested earlier, the analogy was more clearly drawn on one ward than the other. This might have been because staff on Jones Ward had more time to develop the kinds of relationship on which such an analogy might rest, namely 'close' relationships. Alternatively, it might be linked to a different notion of care, as suggested by nurses' different views on 'love' as an element of caring, or the different characteristics of the staff, such as the greater number of male nurses on Smith Ward. The issue of gender is returned to later, but first we will consider how the transformation of the ward into a 'private' or domestic sphere appeared to be effected.

POSTURE AND NORMALISATION

One way in which normalisation was effected on Jones Ward was through nurses' use of gesture and bodily posture. Significantly, it has been claimed that '[to] interpret and account for gesture is to unlock the whole social and cultural system of which it is a part' (Thomas 1991, p.11). It has already been noted that Jones Ward was described as 'relaxed' in a number of respects, such as the way in which nurses planned their work, the lack of rigidity regarding ward 'routine' and the few restraints on patients – creating, in all, a 'homely' as opposed to an institutional atmosphere. In addition, nurses' posture was seen to be very informal. One nurse remarked on this by saying that, as the ward was relaxed in approach, the nurses were relaxed in posture. Nurses were seen to sprawl on the beds (although this particular kind of posture was not encouraged), or very often, when sitting, nurses would tuck their legs up or sit on one leg. It was a common sight to see nurses kneeling on one or both knees while talking to a patient who was in bed or sitting in an armchair. Similarly, one nurse or another would often stand in an exaggerated posture with, for example, legs very wide apart, or sit on the ward desk with her feet on the chair.

Nurses were vaguely aware of their rather unorthodox use of posture. This was suggested to me in the way in which nurses would comment on more formal stances. For example, another nurse and I were made fun of by one of the senior nurses for standing with our arms crossed in a rather traditional nursing pose. During interview, this same nurse commented on the usual posture of nurses:

> You see nurses sitting on patients' beds with their legs curled up, reading the patient's newspaper, going through it with the patient, which if you think about it out of context, then it's an alarming – sort of laid back – thing to do, especially when you think of the age of the person.

She also suggested that nurses' posture was different from that of other occupational groups, saying:

> In an office situation, I couldn't imagine somebody going and perching themselves on someone's desk, putting their feet on the chair, [but here] perching on desks is more of the rule than the exception.

These nurses' posture was, however, different from that of members of their own occupational group, such as the nurses on Smith Ward. While nurses on Smith Ward were informal in their approach, informality was not made visible through stance. This may partly have been because nurses had less space and opportunity to 'lounge about', but this was not the only factor underlying differences between the wards.

Informality could certainly be observed in other forms on Smith Ward. It was evident, for example, in the use of horseplay, the bantering between nurses and between nurses and patients, and in the affection that was expressed towards some patients. However, highly relaxed posture was not encouraged and was regarded by several nurses as 'unprofessional'. One of the senior staff nurses said, for instance:

> I don't like people who feel it's alright to sort of doss around or lounge around when they are at work. I think you should show yourself as a professional person – and I don't think [lounging around] is what the public expects.

In contrast, nurses on Jones Ward thought that relaxed posture was quite consistent with professional behaviour. For example, one primary nurse commented:

> I feel quite comfortable when I'm actually doing nursing squatting on my heels – I feel very comfortable in that unladylike position . . . You see nurses with their hands in their pockets, and talking and discussing and seeming quite relaxed and . . . draping themselves on beds or sitting on the edge of the bed, their legs under them; I don't believe that it's unprofessional. I believe being unprofessional is to do with what you say – it's how you look to a certain extent, but it's to do with your manner, what you say, how you say it.

Female nurses' highly relaxed posture on Jones Ward was usually facilitated by the fact that they wore trousers. Much of their stance would have risked indecency had the nurses been wearing skirts, and the whole meaning of their posture would have been open to a different interpretation. Wearing trousers with a tunic, and sometimes a sweatshirt with the ward logo, also helped in the process of 'normalisation', by reducing the extent to which a nurse looked like a nurse in the traditional sense. For instance, one associate nurse had the following to say about wearing trousers:

> Sitting on beds, you don't have to think about how you are sitting. I know my behaviour is more relaxed with patients, and whether that's to do with the fact

that I've got trousers on ... You're less *nursey* ... you don't feel so restricted ... You're more nursey if you're wearing a dress and have to act in certain ways – to me [being nursey is being] more regimented.

Similarly, one of the primary nurses said:

What strikes me ... is that since we've been wearing trouser suits I feel much more relaxed in the work that I do, and therefore find I put my hands in my pockets and have my sleeves rolled up ... I can see that maybe some people might find it a little unusual if they had a certain idea of what a nurse should look like and how they should act, but I certainly feel a lot more relaxed in trousers.

Nurses on Smith Ward generally had a different approach. Fewer nurses wore trousers, for example. One staff nurse commented that although trousers were more comfortable and more practical, she still felt more 'nursey' in a dress. Although the meaning of this term was not elaborated and may have meant something different for nurses on each ward, it was clear that staff on Jones Ward rejected or resisted feeling and appearing 'nursey', while those nurses who used this term on Smith Ward gave it a more positive gloss. Significantly, the charge nurse was said to disapprove of female staff wearing trousers, and in an interview he said:

It's all got a bit more relaxed since they began to wear trousers and all this business, you see, but whether it's a good thing or a bad thing ... it's hard to say. I mean ... you can be natural or you can be so laid back that you appear like you couldn't give a hoot ... and I sometimes get the impression that, you know, people just stagger in and stagger out, and that looks just as awful as someone being an absolute dictator, strutting, marching about the place.

Asked why nurses might develop a relaxed posture, a number of informants on Jones Ward linked it to the physical nature of nursing; because the nurse's body was central in the provision of care, nurses were accustomed to using the body expressively. However, this does not explain why nurses adopt a relaxed stance on one ward and not on another. While recognising that there may be a range of factors that contribute to this difference, we shall briefly discuss two issues that appear relevant here. These concern the strategic value of redefining the ward as a private space for nurses on Jones Ward, and subtle differences regarding nurses' understandings of nursing itself.

REDRAWING THE PUBLIC:PRIVATE BOUNDARY AS SUBVERSIVE STRATEGY

One part of the explanation for nurses' different posture may lie in the different ratio of male to female nurses on the two wards in the study. It has been suggested that entering Jones Ward, where at any one moment a large proportion of the nurses would be sitting talking to patients, was more like entering the living room in someone's home rather than an institutional space. This sense of the ward as domestic space was endorsed by nurses' use of casual posture. The extent to which this transformation was intentional will be discussed below (see 'Performance'). Before this, however, the potential effects of such a transformation will be considered.

As part of the process of 'normalisation', relaxed posture may help to make the extraordinary easier to cope with by making it more familiar and more reminiscent, not merely of everyday life, but of everyday *private* life. Yet, in contemporary Western culture, this private sphere has been widely associated with what is female (Moore 1988, Sciama 1993). One of the differences between the two wards was that Jones Ward had a predominantly female workforce, while Smith Ward had not only male nurses among the permanent staff, but also a male nurse in overall charge of the ward. This might mean that, because nurses' experience of gender role was differently constituted for each ward, different aims and strategies for providing care emerged.

It has been suggested that, historically, 'nurses have tacitly accepted the stereotyping of their nursing role in the same way as women have accepted stereotyping of female roles' (Street 1992, p. 51). But what appeared to be happening on Jones Ward was that nurses were manipulating stereotypical female roles – or the association between female and private spheres – in order to *challenge* the stereotyping of their nursing role. As Ardener (1993) has said, it is not only important to see how women are prevented from entering certain spaces, but also important to recognise space that women *can* enter and how they may exploit space (see also Spain 1992).

To elaborate, the permanent nurses of Jones Ward – all female – were introducing a new form of nursing which promoted the role of the nurse as an individual practitioner in the face of hostility to change, particularly, as is discussed below, among senior medical colleagues who were all male. Through transforming the context in which they provided nursing care – changing it from a public sphere more closely identified with men to a private sphere where women might have more authority – the nurses appeared to 'pull the rug' from beneath the doctor's feet (to use a nice 'homely' metaphor). Their redefinition of the context of care meant that nurses began to have greater control over the environment in which nursing care took place. Significantly, medical sources reported that, with the new nursing regime, junior doctors were uncomfortable on the ward and stayed away as much as possible.

However, this is not to suggest that nurses had total control over their environment, and, in the face of more senior doctors, the boundary that nurses drew between public and private appeared fairly fragile or unstable, as the following examples indicate.

It has been noted that nurses' posture on Jones Ward was often highly informal. One of the main exceptions to this trend occurred when senior medical staff visited the ward to conduct a ward round. On these occasions, each of the nurses who took turns to accompany the round adopted a stance that was quite different from her usual one. Instead of squatting by the patient's side, slouching in a chair or sitting on the bed, the nurse would stand very straight at the side of the bed, generally with hands crossed behind her back. It was as if the world constructed by the nurses was suspended until the doctors left the ward.

Medical colleagues who arrived on the ward alone or who had not reached consultant status had less impact, and the nurses' definition of space, instead of being instantly overturned, often became the focus of confrontation. For example, nurses had decided that the ward's overhead lights would not be switched on in the morning, to allow patients to wake in their own time rather than being woken according to an institutional regime. This meant that certain tasks, such as giving out breakfasts, were more difficult to perform, particularly in the winter months when parts of the ward remained quite dark until about 8am. The lack of regime, although it appeared to improve the patient's experience of hospitalisation, clearly made life more difficult for staff, and nurses had to work hard to convince others of the benefits. They were generally successful and where they were not, it was generally their medical colleagues who remained unconvinced.[2] Some doctors would make early morning visits to the ward and ask for the lights to be put on. Nurses would usually respond by explaining the policy and suggesting that a patient's bedside light was used instead. On many occasions, doctors would comply. Yet, more than once, one particular doctor, a senior registrar, refused and strode to the main lighting panel to switch on the overhead lights. By this action, it might be argued, through suddenly bathing the whole ward in fluorescent light, he dramatically transformed the ward and reclaimed it as a public space.

The relationship between nurses and doctors is discussed further in Chapter 9. At this point, it is useful to underline the extent to which antagonism between nurses and doctors on Jones Ward was associated with the way its female workforce began to assert their authority through their redefinition, first, of nursing itself as an autonomous discipline, and, subsequently, of the context of nursing, through 'normalising' and 'privatising' the ward. As suggested by the comments of the charge nurse on Smith Ward regarding responsibility for housekeeping, he used a different sort of strategy in his dealings with doctors. His more overtly confrontational style with male doctors may well have been influenced by his gender socialisation.

In interviews, senior doctors expressed less antagonism towards nurses on Smith Ward, which seems largely to be because the style of nursing on Smith Ward had not cut across the interests of doctors to the same extent. For example, generally speaking, the most senior nurse on duty would accompany ward rounds. Thus, the doctor was spared from dealing with junior staff (who were perceived to know less about the patient) and from finding different nurses for different patients. At the same time, there was a sense in which the ward, unlike Jones Ward, remained a public space and was thus more accessible to medical staff. The ward's public nature was maintained by a number of means, including the clear distinction between nurses' and patients' space, the reduced space and opportunity for nurses to sit with patients, and the large number of people visiting the ward at any time. Significantly, junior doctors appeared to spend more time on the ward than on Jones Ward, but their relations with nurses were not noticeably different. On both wards, nurses were not solicitous or coquettish in the way they acted towards doctors. As mentioned above, junior doctors complained that nurses on Smith Ward did not flirt with them like other nurses in the hospital. The different definition of space that seemed to characterise Smith Ward may have been shaped by the fact that the nurse in charge was male, but it also appeared to be influenced by a subtle difference between the two wards concerning the way in which they understood nursing and put this understanding into practice.

TURNING IDEOLOGY INTO PRACTICE

In terms of their perceptions of nursing, nurses on both wards had broadly similar views regarding the need for patients to receive individualised care and the 'rights' of patients concerning equal treatment regardless of ethnic group or creed. Nurses' understanding of 'care' and their commitment to providing high quality care were similar on both wards.

However, while their general philosophy of care was similar, the characteristics of patients differed between the two wards. As stated earlier, patients on Jones Ward were generally chronically ill, while those on Smith Ward were typically older, often acutely ill, and more dependent on nurses for physical care. In addition, nurses faced different constraints in the provision of care; on Smith Ward, for example, they were obliged to spend more time on non-nursing duties because of inadequate numbers of porters (see Chapter 4). Thus, a similar philosophy of care was expressed differently on the two wards because of differences in case mix and in the resources available to nurses.

Moreover, beyond these variables, nurses on the two wards stressed different aspects of nursing and appeared to understand the *process* of nursing in slightly different terms. In some respects, the distinction is described in Chapter 10 in terms of the 'visionary' versus the 'pragmatic' approach identified with each ward. At this point, however, the differences in process that were suggested by nurses' use of their body and spatial relationships, particularly with reference to 'closeness', need to be drawn out.

Jones Ward was a self-designated Nursing Development Unit, with a strong commitment to primary nursing and the concept of a therapeutic relationship between nurse and patient. Nurses, for the most part, expressly wished to develop 'close' relationships with their patients and understood 'closeness' as a core part of nursing care. On Smith Ward, although the notion of 'closeness' was understood in a similar way and positively valued, it was not as central to the actual provision of care. Although this distinction may have been linked to a different view of nursing – nurses on Smith Ward gave rather less stress to the therapeutic potential of nursing as it is defined by the 'new nursing' movement – it was also clearly associated with the lack of resources available to nurses on Smith Ward; it needs to be stressed that nurses were often frustrated in their attempts to provide the kind of care they wished to give. In contrast, Jones Ward was well resourced, and nurses were generally able to practise at a level at which there was a close correspondence between aims and practice.

For nurses on Jones Ward, it appeared that one way of developing and demonstrating 'closeness' was through the use of physical proximity. In many situations, this close physical presence might have been misinterpreted, but by redefining the context in which it occurred – by transforming the ward into a domestic space where physical nearness takes on a different meaning – nurses were able to put their philosophy regarding 'closeness' into practice. They could make evident their wish to share the patient's physical and emotional space through their use of the body.

Nurses' adoption of casual and 'open' posture (with legs, for example, wide apart) can also be seen as an inversion of the stance generally expected of women in the public domain. Women often use smaller and less open bodily movements than men when in public, keeping their arms close to their body and their legs together (Wex 1979). 'Openness' in women might be interpreted as a sign of weakness or loose moral conduct (Creyghton 1982). Alternatively, a posture that is more 'closed' may arise, at least in part, from the threat of physical invasion that women constantly experience (rape being the most extreme form); women tend to construct a barrier around themselves through their use of bodily stance, to keep others at a distance and to protect themselves from invasion (Young 1990). As is quoted elsewhere (Savage 1991), without denying the harsh reality of some women's domestic lives, this barrier is generally dismantled in the domestic sphere where 'openness' begins to take on a more positive value (as in consensual sexual intercourse, for example).

In contrast, the posture of men does not vary as much between public and private spheres. It is, nonetheless, influenced by context – for example, in groups of men, those with high status will adopt a looser and more relaxed stance than their juniors (Bartky 1988). If we take posture as an indictor of power or status, the typical bodily language of women in the public domain, 'a language of relative tension and constriction' (Bartky 1988, p.73), can be seen as a language of subordination. It is, therefore, easy to imagine how female nurses' relaxed or open posture – a stance that denies subordination – might antagonise their male medical colleagues, yet hold a very different meaning for their patients.

On Jones Ward, it appears that transforming the context from public to private allowed female nurses to be 'open' or receptive to their patients. In the discussion of metaphor earlier, we saw how the effect of 'closeness' was to allow the patient (and possibly the nurse) to 'open up', and how this 'opening up' seemed to lie at the heart of the therapeutic relationship. It is possible that this 'openness', like 'closeness', may be expressed physically by nurses, in this instance through their open stance, in a way that runs counter to a mind–body dualism. As we saw before, such embodiment of nursing aims can also be glimpsed in the way in which nurses on Jones Ward spoke of their desire to empower their patients and foster equality and, correspondingly, adopted positions, such as squatting by the patient's side, that placed them 'at the patient's level'.

On Smith Ward, however, 'closeness', 'openness' and 'parity' with the patient were not acted out in the same way; Smith Ward was a far more 'public' space than its counterpart, with correspondingly 'public' stances adopted by the female staff. This appears to be partly because of its staff's different perceptions of the process of nursing or how nursing 'works'. For example, besides less stress on the therapeutic nature of 'closeness', there was less non-spontaneous use of expressive touch (or touch for the sake of touch), which, on Jones Ward, appeared to demonstrate and reinforce 'closeness'. In addition, there was clearly a different attitude towards the adoption of relaxed posture by nurses (as shown, for example, by the charge nurse's comments on 'dossing around', see above).

In this and earlier sections, it has been suggested that nurses on Jones Ward embodied or, alternatively, 'played out' elements of nursing philosophy, such as 'closeness', 'openness' or 'parity' and that this suggested a certain kind of knowledge. This knowledge held by nurses was concerned with how they might use their own physicality in the therapeutic process that is the 'new nursing'. (The issue of whether or how the effectiveness of this therapy can be evaluated is not considered here.)

The apparent existence of this knowledge raises a number of interesting questions. For example, to what extent is such knowledge embodied and, thus, not consciously initiated, and to what degree are nurses' physical actions (their coming 'close', their use of touch, their posture) informed by conscious intent and, by implication, representing some kind of performance?

PERFORMANCE

In this section, we will briefly examine the extent to which it is helpful to look at nurses' actions on the two wards as kinds of performance. It is hoped that this approach will be useful in further exploring nurses' manipulation of symbolic space and what this manipulation can tell us about non-verbal nursing knowledge.

Goffman (1971) has drawn an analogy between actions staged in a theatre and the structure of everyday encounters. He claims that (p.246):

> [the] key factor in this structure is the maintenance of a *single definition of the situation*, this definition having to be expressed, and this definition sustained, in the face of a multitude of potential disruptions.

Settings of health-care provision or institutional care, such as hospitals, are characterised by ambiguity. We have already seen, for example, how nurses' intimate involvement with patients requiring physical care transgresses the usual 'rules' governing behaviour between relative strangers. Nurses (and patients – see for instance Emerson 1971) have to manage this ambiguity and define which of a number of possible definitions of reality underlie their actions. Weiss (1993), in a study of behaviour on grand rounds in an Israeli teaching hospital, shows how the definition of reality can be made clear through the use of drama. Weiss observes that contact with excreta and organic process is generally associated with personnel of low status, yet this is often a necessary aspect of physicians' work. The way in which doctors deal with this paradox on rounds is either by concealing their involvement – to protect themselves against imputed 'pollution' – or by restating their status through the grand round, which is presented as a form of performance, with a fixed script, standard costumes and routinised behaviour, including joking of a chauvinistic or sexist nature. According to Weiss, the connection between the grand round and drama and the stage is more than simple artifice; with the creation of a theatrical setting, everyday reality is masked and a distance is created between the hospital and the real world. Weiss (1993, p.250) concludes:

> By making their socially disapproved acts dramatic, they enable themselves to appear to be on stage, actors acting out an imaginary role that is in no way connected with their real selves. Grand rounds thus protect the actors against threats to status, while at the same time actively asserting that status.[3]

In line with the argument that nurses on the two wards drew a different boundary between public and private in their 'single definition of the situation', it was more common for nurses on Smith Ward to emphasise a distinction between their behaviour at home and at work, or to imply that their behaviour at work was a form of performance. As the charge nurse said:

> I think people out of work are very different to when they're in work. I mean, I am ... I'm totally and absolutely different when I'm at work. It's a false part actually; it's just like two different characters in some ways.

Similarly, one of the staff nurses said of her colleagues on the ward:

yes, they're good friends, [but] nurses are very strange in that way – they'd be shocked seeing me outside work. I mean, I'm still quite sort of lively, chatty and that, but you're just different. [It's] the same with everybody. Of course, you're different; you've got to be different in different situations, especially on here.

Thus, there was something about Smith Ward that meant that nurses were 'acting out an imaginary role that is in no way connected with their real selves' (Weiss 1993, p.250). Quite what this was can only be speculated. For instance, in the context of Weiss's analysis, it is interesting that nurses on Smith Ward were more involved than those on Jones Ward in what has been termed 'dirty work' (Douglas 1966, Lawler 1991). Their clear separation between their working and non-working selves might, therefore, be linked to the ambiguity of their status as a result of being 'intimately involved and identified with the containment of personal pollution' (Littlewood 1991, p.178).

In contrast, nurses on Jones Ward often gave the impression that there was very little difference between their management of the self on and off duty. As one associate nurse put it:

The barriers between your working role and your social role are possibly broken down a bit more [in this ward]; there's more of *me* – the outside me – in the working environment.

This corresponded with other comments nurses made about being less 'nursey' than on Smith Ward. It was as if, by defining the ward's space as 'home', there was no necessity for – or possibility of – drawing a distinction between who they were at work and who they were 'outside'. However, it should be remembered that nurses did not have to manage 'reality' in quite the same way as did nurses on Smith Ward; for example, 'dirty work' was not a constant feature of care.

This is not to suggest, however, that a clear distinction can be made between the style of nursing on the two wards, with nurses on one ward giving a kind of performance and those on the other ward behaving 'naturally' or as they would in any other context – in other words, that one group of nurses are 'false' and calculating and the other sincere. For one thing, 'behaviour and space are mutually dependent' (Ardener 1993, p. 2): social identity is always partly determined by the physical and spatial aspects of people's environment, implying that identity is always context dependent. Instead, it seems that features of the two wards were such that, overall, they demanded different 'presentations of self' (Goffman 1971). As we have seen, these 'features' are complex, including, for example, the ward's case mix and physical layout, the resources available to staff, the attitudes of other health workers and the gender socialisation of the nurses.

As Ersser (1991) has pointed out, much of the previous analysis of social interactions (such as Goffman's work relating to 'deep' and 'surface' acting), as well as work on the therapeutic use of self (for example Travelbee 1971) or nurses' emotional labour (Smith 1992), has been primarily concerned with the *deliberate* management of appearances or emotions, yet we cannot assume that nurses' emotional interaction with patients is always a product of conscious intent. While the development of emotional 'closeness' between nurses and patients is assumed to allow opportunities for therapeutic intervention, 'the effective use of such opportunities in a way that, at the very least, does not do more harm than good requires tremendous skill on the part of nurses' (Ersser 1991, p.66). We have already identified some of these skills, represented, for example, by nurses' use of body posture and humour. At this point, therefore, it is worth considering the way in which these skills are deployed in terms of whether they are consciously or unconsciously applied.

CONSCIOUSNESS

Nurses on both wards were aware of being performers at some level. For example, they referred to how they tended to walk in a different way – usually more quickly – once they had crossed the ward's threshold. Alternatively, in certain circumstances, nurses might deliberately convey a sense of speed and urgency in order to reduce patients' expectations regarding care or any opportunity for conversation. In particular, those in the study frequently referred to 'strutting' as a general characteristic of nurses. During fieldwork, both 'speeding' and 'strutting' were more commonly observed on Smith Ward than Jones Ward. As the charge nurse said:

> I enjoy, actually, to be frank, having a bit of influence – there's an element of power that I do enjoy . . . I remember going into a bay one day and strutting in and saying, 'Good afternoon gentlemen!' – very sort of formal – and someone said it was like meeting the Prince of Wales or something; there's that sort of strutting that goes on.

This self-awareness was echoed by another nurse from Smith Ward, who said:

> If I move very rapidly around the ward it could be [that] I'm feeling annoyed about something . . . or that I've got a lot to get done . . . It's something that I'm very conscious of – how I move around the ward.

Nurses also spoke of how, if they wanted to encourage a patient to talk, they might indicate this by sitting down or adopting a position similar to that of the patient. This was not necessarily something they were aware of doing in advance, but 'maybe halfway through, you'd notice'. At the same time, nurses were aware of being observed by patients, which heightened their sense of putting on a performance. For example, one of the primary nurses on Jones Ward said:

> I think you are a performer in that [patients] watch you, and they know so much about you, because they are there 24 hours a day . . . so in that respect, I suppose you are on show.

Several nurses commented on the way in which subgroups of nurses might develop a certain style in common. Some informants, for instance, referred to how easy it was to recognise nurses from the A&E department (when this still existed) if they were seen elsewhere in the hospital, but hard to explain why they were so recognisable. It was not only that they carried stethoscopes; these nurses also wore their uniform in ways that were subtly different from those of other nurses, and most notably they had a characteristic stance. Thus, it seems that the identification of a certain kind of posture with a particular kind of specialty or unit extended beyond the wards in the study.

According to Okely (1992, p.17), during participant observation, 'the fieldworker both consciously and unconsciously responds to certain rhythms and patterns as immersion proceeds'. During her research among Traveller Gypsies, a photograph of Okely and a Traveller woman was taken by a stranger. Okely notes how in this photograph she has 'unknowingly imitated the Gypsy woman's defensive bodily posture'. The posture in question is one of standing with weight evenly distributed between both feet, with arms crossed and head slightly turned away from the camera. Her comments are of interest of two reasons. First, Okely indicates something of the way in which shared posture is taken up 'unknowingly' by people who share their lives in some regular manner. A similar point has been made by Mauss (1973), who observed how those of the same gender or social class, or people in similar employment, come to share similar 'techniques of the body' as a result of their shared social environment.

Second, the posture to which Okely refers is similar to one that nurses used to adopt. Writing on interpersonal relationships in 1979, for example, Burton referred to the way in which nurses kept their arms crossed throughout many of their interactions. In common with many of my peers, I remember adopting a similar stance, in which my arms would be tucked behind the bib of my starched apron. As I recall, this pose was adopted by a large number of nurses, both qualified and in training. Together with a few other relatively relaxed poses that we were able to adopt in the absence of more senior nurses, it seemed to represent a statement about group identity and a rejection of the formal stance that nurses were expected to take in their work.[4] The pose itself differed from that described by Okely; it felt, as I remember, more relaxed than defensive. However, it was clearly not an 'open' stance, as characterised by nurses on Jones Ward. As mentioned above, I became aware during the current fieldwork that this traditional pose of crossed arms had largely disappeared, at least among those nurses who had adopted the 'new nursing'.

Interestingly, nurses I spoke to seemed half aware of the postures they adopted. For example, one of the senior nurses on Jones Ward showed that she was on occasions aware of her stance when she said:

> I think I use my body in different ways in different situations. If I'm doing a ward round – which I don't do very often – I'm aware that I stand with my hands behind my back, and I don't usually have any interaction with the patient during the ward round. I will go and stand or sit by the patient, but there's not a lot of communication that goes on in that way.

An associate nurse on Jones Ward was once observed in conversation with an elderly, frail patient; the nurse was kneeling on the floor, at the side of his chair, with her face close to the patient's and her arms resting on the chair arm. The overall effect was to suggest a filial relationship or, more accurately, one between a grandfather and granddaughter, a storytelling or an exchange of confidences. Talking to the nurse later, I referred to this episode and asked whether she was aware of the effect created by her body language or whether her use of such language was subconscious. She replied:

> It's probably a mixture of the two, I think. I mean, it's something that I'm aware of, in that it is nicer for the person, but I generally do it without thinking about it . . . I don't particularly concentrate on whether I've got my arms crossed or my legs crossed or if I am looking defensive.

Significantly, this nurse was not alone among nurses on Jones Ward in commenting that her bodily attitude was similar at home and at work. Yet this does not necessarily mean that such behaviour was entirely spontaneous or uninformed by any intent. For instance, after several months 'in the field', I forgot my initial impressions regarding nurses' behaviour, but my fieldnotes show that I originally felt that nurses' use of non-instrumental touch was unspontaneous. This was especially clear during the handover, when there was a marked degree of self-consciousness on the part of nurses and patients regarding the nature of the process, including how nurses arranged themselves around the patient or how they used touch. This self-consciousness could, of course, have been intensified by the presence of a researcher, but, as we saw in the section on touch in Chapter 7, nurses' behaviour, especially during the handover, had been described as 'false' by some nurses who were not permanently attached to the ward. I certainly felt awkward when I initially joined nurses on the handover and tried to find ways of positioning myself that fitted in with everyone else's behaviour but which felt comfortable to me. Yet as I spent more time on the ward, I experienced a change in my use of touch and posture, which began to match those of the permanent staff, yet still felt comfortable and largely spontaneous to me. However, I became more cognisant of this process than did the nurses on the ward, because of my research focus.

In terms of understanding how nurses develop an embodied knowledge that helps them to develop particular types of relationships with patients and to clarify the nature of these relationships, I should point out that nurses on Jones Ward were explicitly encouraged to adopt certain postures – such as ensuring that during most interactions they were at a patient's eye level rather than looming over him. Nurses new to the ward, for example, were instructed to use certain forms of stance, such as squatting beside the patient. Yet there was *also* a way in which learning occurred implicitly rather than explicitly and stemmed from emulation, kinaesthetic awareness and observation rather than formal instruction. This implicit knowledge was not simply a matter of imitation. As my own experience on both wards suggested, shared gestures and stance represented a developing understanding of the practical constraints that nurses faced (such as the physical characteristics of the ward or the power relations that operated there) and, in addition, of the principles that helped to shape the ward's style of nursing. So, for example, nurses on Jones Ward came to know through observation and lived experience that they could use 'open' informal posture in the presence of nurse managers but not in their dealings with senior medical colleagues. Similarly, these nurses 'knew', without formal instruction, that gestures reminiscent of the domestic sphere were appropriate for the development of their relationships with patients, just as nurses on Smith Ward 'knew' at some level that these same gestures were inappropriate for the form of nursing they practised or the context in which they worked. In this way, nurses' bodily practices can be seen to 'mediate a personal realisation of social values' (Jackson 1983, p.337); such values become 'known' and expressed through the body.

ENDNOTES

1. 'Somology' is a term introduced by Lawler to refer to an understanding of the body that takes into account that the body is simultaneously 'an object, a means of experience, a means of expression, a manner of presence among other people, and a part of one's personal identity' (1991, p.29).
2. More accurately, it was doctors who were perhaps in a position to hold out against change; some of the domestic staff were unenthusiastic about the lack of lighting early in the morning, but nurses were usually able to overrule such objections because of their greater authority on the ward.
3. For a more detailed discussion of performance see, for example, Goffman (1971), Schechner (1990) and Bell (1992).
4. This refers to the late 1960s when, as student nurses, we were expected to

rearrange our dress – to remove 'frillies', roll down our sleeves and put on starched cuffs – before addressing senior staff, such as the ward sister. We were also expected to stand when doctors entered the office or open doors for senior doctors and let them pass first. It is in this context that standing with arms folded behind an apron bib can be described as 'relaxed'.

9

The Support Needs of Nurses

So far, we have explored what the notion of 'closeness' means to nurses and the ways in which they foster and express 'closeness'. In this chapter, we will return to one of the original questions that shaped the research, namely, what are the implications for nurses if they are encouraged to develop 'close' relationships with patients? Are nurses who practise the 'new nursing' highly stressed or do they find ways of sustaining 'close' relationships with patients without incurring great personal cost?

First, this chapter will present the views of nurses on both wards regarding the support they received, the forms this support may have assumed and the kinds of initiative they believed would help to sustain them in their work. The final section then examines the relationship between the features of the different wards, including the different nursing styles they adopted, the support needs of nurses and the general context in which the nursing took place.

JONES WARD

According to the senior nurse manager, Jones Ward had a low staff turnover rate, especially among more senior staff, and a low sickness rate (about 2%). She thought that this was, to a certain extent, explained by the supportive nature of relationships on the ward. Significantly, the reciprocal nature of nurse–patient relations was evident to this manager as, under the rubric of 'support for nurses', she explicitly included the sympathy and concern that patients expressed for the nurses who cared for them.

However, the support available from colleagues and patients is not necessarily the only explanation for a low incidence of staff sickness and turnover; rates were very similar for most wards in the hospital where Jones Ward was located. One possible explanation for this similarity might lie in the wider changes occurring within the health authority and beyond. Widespread ward closures, uncertainty about attempts to rationalise health care services, as well as doubts about which hospitals could successfully compete in the new market economy, all meant that staff had fewer employment options and were tending to stay longer in post. In addition, because all posts were being scrutinised, with many nurses being asked to reapply for their own position, staff everywhere were reluctant to diminish their chances of being retained by having a poor health record. Thus, ostensibly objective measures, such as staff turnover and sickness rates, were not reliable indicators that staff were well supported or that morale was high.

Matters were no clearer from a subjective perspective. Particularly towards the end of the research period, when the rate of change was rapidly accelerating throughout hospitals in the area, there was little in the nurses' everyday demeanour to indicate the inner turmoil many of them must have been experiencing. Their skills as 'performers' (see Chapter 8) seemed to include the ability to conceal distress resulting from rapid change and seemingly endless restructuring. Just as nurses 'coped' admirably with the harsh realities they were exposed to in their everyday practice, they appeared, for the most part, adroit at concealing any stress they experienced in the face of job insecurity, loss of resources or role change.

On the basis of data derived from interviews, it appeared that nurses' support needs were not straightforward. Many apparently contradictory statements were made by informants about the extent and the nature of the support they required. Several nurses, for example, claimed that they felt adequately supported by colleagues but then, at a later point in the discussion, said that they would appreciate the services of a counsellor or would otherwise hint that their support needs were greater than first intimated. Other nurses referred to the stressful nature of nursing but said that they had little personal need of support.

Besides the possibility that nurses were unwilling to discuss their problems with the researcher, or to acknowledge a growing inability to cope, one of the main explanations for these apparent contradictions seems to lie in the range of situations that nurses find themselves in and the speed with which their environment can change. Hence, nurses who spoke of feeling adequately supported on one occasion might feel very differently on another. In addition, there was a wide range of situations in which nurses thought support would be needed but indicated that they did not experience this need themselves. What was significant was that, in response to a question referring to nurses' support needs without specifying the area of need, only a few nurses spontaneously referred to the nature of the nurse–patient relationship as an area of concern.

Among the nurses interviewed, not one informant referred to the implications of 'closeness'. Instead, these nurses spoke of a generalised stress that was experienced in relation to patients and their illnesses, much as Menzies (1970) has described (see Chapter 2). For example, one primary nurse described a sense of acute, almost permanent grief that she and other nurses felt for patients who were ill, so much so that it became difficult for nurses to accept their own personal troubles or anxieties as legitimate concerns in the face of the greater problems experienced by their patients. Although this tendency to reject their own needs was well recognised by senior nurses within the hospital, such an acknowledgement did little, of itself, to decrease the stress that nurses experienced. A number of nurses thought that a counsellor attached to each unit might be of help. This 'almost permanent grief', however, was not seen as specific to organisational modes, such as primary nursing, or the 'close' relationships that might ensue with continuity of care.

Echoing the comments of the senior nurse manager regarding sources of support, one primary nurse firmly objected to the suggestion that nurses using primary nursing should, *ipso facto*, need more support; this was to imply that a close relationship with a patient was generally likely to have negative consequences for a nurse, yet this was not the case:

> While you do have a close relationship with patients, that doesn't necessarily mean that you are more likely to be stressed out. Conversely, it may be more supportive to feel that you have more of a close relationship with patients.

The three primary nurses tended to refer less to their own need for support than to the needs of more junior nurses who, they believed, might have difficulty coping with a more intense nurse–patient relationship because of inexperience. However, neither associate nurses nor student nurses gave the nature of the nurse–patient relationship as a reason for requiring further support. Similarly, one of the senior nurses thought that the primary nurses had the greatest need of support, facing greater expectations not only from patients, but also from management and junior staff. Yet all three primary nurses, when interviewed, stated that they generally felt adequately supported in their work. They recognised that they had greater responsibilities than other nurses on the ward, but, in general, they felt that their greater experience helped them to cope with this. It is, however, clearly significant that, 18 months after the end of this study, not one of these primary nurses remained in post, despite their previous long association with the ward. This point will be returned to later.

When nurses *were* in need of support they said that they tended to turn to their peers. However, who was regarded as a peer was not always self-evident. Different nurses appeared to turn to different colleagues on different occasions, suggesting that the demarcation between groups of nurses was fluid. The way in which primary nursing fragmented the ward staff into three 'teams' was seen by some nurses to make it more difficult to find appropriate support, if required. This fragmentation was exacerbated by the lack of a specific nursing space, such as an office, in which peers from across the groups could meet as a matter of course. In contrast, other nurses stated that they readily found support either within their group or across groups, as need and circumstances dictated. As one D grade nurse said:

> I think we all support each other at work. If there are any problems, we talk to each other and get it out of our system that way . . . We all work together really.

One or two nurses suggested that less experienced, and thus more vulnerable, staff were more visible working in small groups and were, therefore, less likely to get 'lost' or stressed without others noticing than was the case with other organisational modes.

Significantly, an older and highly experienced associate nurse felt that support was not always available inasmuch as she preferred to turn to staff of her own age if in need. She commented on the way that permanent staff formed two distinct age groups. Nurses of 30 years or more fell into one group, while the other comprised nurses in their early 20s (see Chapter 3, Table 1). Thus, for this nurse at least, the ward was 'fractured' by age as well as nursing groups. Sociocultural categories such as class, gender or ethnic group were not referred to.

During ward meetings on Jones Ward attended during the study, there was some discussion of the need for a regular, possibly multidisciplinary, support group or a regular session with a psychotherapist. It appeared that the idea of introducing this form of support was to help staff cope with specific circumstances that arose rather than the ongoing demands of nurse–patient interaction. Many nurses responded to the suggestion of regular sessions with a counsellor or psychotherapist with ambivalence. It was suggested that support was generally needed on an immediate basis and could not wait for a formalised support session. A number of nurses also commented on the way in which formal support sessions did little to relieve stress and had the potential of making nurses feel more vulnerable; again linking with the discussion on performance or 'front', staff were concerned that innermost conflicts and emotions might be revealed, but to little practical effect. This would make them feel worse.

If 'closeness' with patients did not seem to create specific support needs for nurses, there were other aspects of nurses' work arising from or associated with primary nursing that did lead to stress. Student nurses, for example, felt secure when working with their primary nurse or another, more experienced, associate nurse. However, if they were the only nurse on duty for their group of patients, this forced them into certain situations, such as dealing with medical consultants on ward rounds, for which they often felt unprepared. A number of nurses also referred to the unease they experienced working in a small group and not knowing what was happening beyond this, although this usually became less of a problem the longer the nurse worked on the ward.

Nurses' relationships with medical staff were also a source of stress in a more general sense. As indicated above, the consultants attached to the wards were, on the whole, not in favour of primary nursing and were resistant to many of the changes that nurses wished to introduce as a result of rethinking their nursing practice. This meant, for example, that although the ward was a Nursing Development Unit, with staff committed to research-based practice, highly experienced nurses were routinely prevented from carrying out nursing procedures such as the changing of dressings. Despite their stress on partnership with patients, or the empowerment of patients, nurses were often thwarted in carrying through changes that helped to alter the ward's ambiance and make it more oriented towards patients' requirements, as the above example of the ward lights has illustrated.

A further form of stress occurred at weekends when staffing levels dropped but the number of time-consuming procedures (such as the administration of intravenous drugs) increased. Following a district-wide agreement to take over certain tasks from junior doctors, nurses often had to change groups at weekends in order to allow a suitably qualified member of staff to give intravenous medications. This led to discontinuity of care and lack of knowledge about patients. Thus, rather than finding that continuity of care and the 'close' relationships developed through primary nursing led to stress for nurses, it seemed that stress occurred when the primary nursing system disintegrated due to staff shortages and nurses were prevented from *maintaining* the relationships they had established with patients.

SMITH WARD

On Smith Ward, nurses' support needs took a clearer form; for the most part, nurses experienced stress as a result of being unable to provide the kind of care they wished to give their patients. There were two particular sources of stress. First, in the midst of a busy surgical ward, there was a group of patients for whom only palliative treatment was available and who were often terminally ill. These patients had particular psychological as well as physical needs, yet nurses felt they had insufficient time or skills to offer this group appropriate care. There were no counsellors available within the hospital to assist patients, relatives or staff, and nurses from the ward experienced great difficulty in obtaining further training in this area. As one senior staff nurse said:

> We desperately need a counsellor but can't afford to get one . . . I think it's a very sad lack in the hospital. I mean, there's nobody when you have bereaved relatives – sometimes extremely distressed relatives. Number one: you haven't the facilities to cope with them. Number two: we haven't got the skills. Number three: we haven't got the time. I think it's a big lack, particularly as we have the

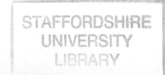

laser patients – it's a palliative treatment [for cancer of the oesophagus], and it's a known fact that once [patients] start coming for laser, the longest they live is a year and a half. That's the very longest. The average is nine months, and you see them coming in and gradually deteriorating, and it's sad – that's all I can say – that [counselling] is not seen to be a priority. It's a shame.

Second, the hospital as a whole and, within it, Smith Ward, was under-resourced. In addition to two D grade posts that were frozen, the senior nurse manager for the ward estimated that it required two further nurses of D grade to alleviate the chronic overload that nurses experienced. The charge nurse made a similar point, referring to the:

lack of staff, heavy patient workload, frustration in not being able to do the job that you know you can do . . . I think it's the same throughout the hospital, probably in every department that, you know, there just aren't enough people to do the job that they've got to do.

One example of this widespread shortage related to an insufficient number of hospital porters and other ancillary staff. A particular consequence of this was that nurses carried out a large number of non-nursing duties or spent an inordinate amount of time trying to organise support services.

Nurses were frustrated in their ability to provide good nursing care, not only by shortages of staff, but also by the lack of patient privacy resulting from cramped conditions. The environment was poor, in that the ward needed painting and general upgrading. The layout not only made continuity of care difficult, but also meant that it was extremely difficult for nurses to organise their work and to observe all their patients as they would wish. As the charge nurse said, 'The more complex the geography, the more difficult it gets'.

In addition, it was noted by one or two nurses that, partly because of the ward's specialty, non-NHS sources of funding were not available to counterbalance shortfalls in NHS provision; gastroenterology was not as emotive as, for example, paediatrics or oncology. Nor did the hospital have large endowment funds to buffer the shortages that the wards experienced.

The ward had suffered as a result of the long-term absence of a senior nurse manager due to sickness, but there was resentment towards senior management more generally:

I don't feel supported by nursing management. Their nursing has gone out the window. I think that on the ward, the support we get here is great. I don't think there's ever been a moment where I haven't felt supported by the team that I work with on the ward . . . but I don't feel supported by nursing management. (Associate nurse)

As with nurses on Jones Ward, staff worked in the midst of great change and uncertainty, which was obviously stressful in itself. One or two informants commented on the unenviable position of nurses and others in middle management and were well aware of the constraints they faced. However, it was thought that nurse managers and others needed to listen more closely to those in clinical practice. As one associate nurse said:

[What] I feel frustrated about most is that nobody seems to listen to . . . the nurses that are working on the wards. The message is just not getting through to whoever it needs to go to, you know, that we just haven't got enough staff, we haven't got the resources. You know, we are killing ourselves every day here.

More could also be done to acknowledge the achievements of ward-level nurses. As one nurse said, 'They have the complaints procedure, but they don't actually have the opposite of that – a procedure that actually extends to people praising our care'.

The role of the ward sister or charge nurse was seen as particularly difficult; although credited as the linchpin of the organisation, she or he was seen, in reality, as 'the piggy in the middle' who was 'fired on from all directions'. On Smith Ward, the charge nurse was seen to offer support to staff, but it was not clear whether he himself received support. He said that seniority did not, in itself, imply an ability to offer support in all situations, and it was important to be able to admit when one was out of one's depth. However, what facilities were available for those charge nurses or sisters who felt out of their depth was not clear.

Nurses on Smith Ward also referred to the lack of support from medical colleagues. Tensions between medical and nursing staff were not as overt as on Jones Ward, perhaps because the organisational mode was one that doctors were more familiar with and one that challenged them less. During the period of fieldwork, for example, there was still one identifiable nurse coordinator, often the most senior nurse on duty, who would be available for the entirety of a ward round.

However, just as on Jones Ward, doctors' perceptions of nursing were considerably different from nurses', and nursing care often appeared to be judged on the basis of how well nurses assisted doctors, rather than by the standard of patient care they offered. The perception of nurses as housekeepers was referred to in Chapter 4. In addition, nurses resented the way they were expected to 'mother' junior doctors to ensure that they carried out all their tasks. As one nurse said, 'If *nurses* had to be continually reminded to do their job, they'd be disciplined'. On the other hand, if nurses were struggling to lift heavy patients, doctors and medical students would stand and watch, without offering to help. Similarly, after procedures such as venesection, medical staff would leave any mess they made for nurses to clear up.

Moreover, nurses' observations about their patients would be ignored or given little weight. A house officer was overheard to praise the new registrar because of the way he took what was said by the nurse on the ward round 'with a pinch of salt'. Nurses on both wards expressed difficulty in getting junior house officers to visit patients they were concerned about, especially if observations of blood pressure and pulse were equivocal; the nurse's personal knowledge of the patient counted for nothing. As one nurse said of doctors in general, 'They don't understand what we do'.

Smith Ward was very similar to Jones Ward in terms of staff turnover and sickness rates. Of course, although nurses were located in different hospitals, their mobility was subject to similar restrictions, such as the shrinking job market. Nonetheless, the acting nurse manager perceived the permanent work force on Smith Ward as stable and thought that they had found their own ways of coping with the nature and demands of the ward. However, sickness rates for student nurses were slightly higher than for permanent staff, and it was recognised by the nurse manager and permanent ward staff alike that when the ward was busy (as it always was), the needs of the students suffered.

This aside, the comments of students and trained staff suggested that they all found a high degree of support among members of the ward team. Most commonly, nurses referred to the way in which the senior staff nurses and the charge nurse could 'pick up' when nurses were under stress. The nature of much day-to-day support, however, was often unspoken. Nurses sensed that their colleagues were troubled through non-verbal cues, such as 'how they looked'. Similarly, nurses often gained support non-verbally:

> I don't think people necessarily have to say anything. You know when people are [noticing]; you can *feel* support. If you're in an environment where there is none, you're really aware of it. I think we've got a good combination here. There's very good support here, but I don't think it's anything tangible; I think it's just there. And should the need for it ever arise, then it would be there, more measurably. (Senior staff nurse)

This suggests a parallel between the kind of understanding nurses might develop with their patients as described in the 'new nursing' literature, an understanding that often appears to be expressed through the body or through 'being with' the patient, and nurses' understanding of their peers, which is also gained and expressed non-verbally.

Support was not only non-verbal, however, and the value of 'having a rant' or a 'moan' was commented on by a number of nurses. Break times were used 'to let off steam', and the charge nurse's office was often the place where this occurred. As one staff nurse said:

> I usually just go into the office and have a bloody good moan. I tend to find that if you're having a moan, someone else will join in; it's great to get it out in the open.

When problems were aired, these were often expressed in a humorous way. This underlines the points made in Chapter 7 about humour; Coser (1960) has observed, for example, that humour can help to reduce social distance and relax the rigidity of a social structure. It can provide a means of asking for and giving support, and of affirming common values where there is ambiguity or uncertainty. Again, as with normalisation or the appropriate use of touch, the skills required to shape a context through strategies such as humour represent an important element of nurses' work, which may be a highly fruitful area for further investigation. Perhaps because of their use of humour as a means of offering support, coping with uncertainty and managing social relationships, Smith Ward was widely regarded as 'a very happy ward', despite the nature of the work and the lack of resources.

Like nurses on Jones Ward, most permanent staff did not favour formal support groups as an appropriate way of alleviating the stress they experienced. This was partly because when support was required, it represented an immediate need. However, there were those, like the charge nurse, who felt that there was some place for a support group:

> Support may be needed by the group of nurses as a whole and not just on an individual basis. For this reason, I feel outside support from someone who is not emotionally involved in the situation would be a more sensible way of being more fully objective and able to identify the core issues.

Yet, sadly, many nurses saw that the core issues were linked to a poor level of resources. This meant that most solutions were beyond their control, and thus support groups would be ineffective. As one staff nurse said, 'If resources were more adequate, we'd have less need of support'.

To summarise, nurses on both wards, irrespective of organisational mode or perceptions of nursing, developed support systems integral to the ward team. The support offered on this basis was often tacit in nature, yet played a significant role in sustaining nurses in their everyday practice. The stability of both ward teams and the length of time nurses had worked together appeared to be important factors in the development of this informal support. Contrary to the initial expectations of the study, 'close' relationships with patients were generally not experienced as a source of stress; indeed, they could be a source of support. Rather, it was relationships with health personnel outside the ward team, particularly medical staff, that were problematic. Lack of awareness of what nurses do – or what nursing is – undermined nurses' ability to use their skills fully or develop their potential. This permanent constraint on nurses, in itself, constituted a form of stress. As we have seen in Chapter 8, nurses did not passively accept this situation but developed strategies that, for example, challenged the distribution of power between nurses and their medical colleagues. These strategies were not always successful. However, what appeared more stressful to nurses, perhaps because they had no hope of overcoming the problem, was the distress they experienced when they were unable to offer the standard of care they aspired to give, because of the lack of a whole range of resources. This point will be taken up again in Chapter 10.

THE NATURE OF THE WARD TEAM

One final point is linked to the support available to nurses and is also of more general relevance. It concerns the relationship between ward ideology and the nature of the nursing team. For example, one staff nurse on Smith Ward commented, in relation to the informal support he received from colleagues:

> I feel . . . relaxed with the staff [on this ward] and it amazes me . . . that you can get such a nice mix of people as, you know, there's no rule to say that you all have to like each other.

There were many differences between nurses on each ward in terms of their social backgrounds, experience or personalities, yet each ward team also had a distinctive style or ethos. This may be very loosely expressed in terms of the 'visionary' nature of the nurses' approach on Jones Ward and the 'pragmatic' nature of that on Smith Ward. This ward style appeared to be largely created by the senior ward staff in terms of their everyday practice and their priorities when recruiting new staff.

During interviews, statements from more junior staff occasionally gave glimpses of the way in which their senior colleagues provided role models (see for example Chapter 6). In addition, senior staff had specific characteristics that they looked for in potential recruits who already met the standard requirements of the job description. These characteristics were different for each ward and helped to explain the specific character of each ward team.

For Jones Ward, it was important that new nurses were interested in nursing issues and committed to the development of nursing and the aims of the ward team. In this respect, those recruiting new staff looked for similar characteristics in candidates for both primary and associate nurse posts. Linked to this, all nurses needed to have given some thought to nurse accountability, although in practice this would have different implications for primary and associate nurses. Associate nurses had to be able 'to cope with being directed' and open to questioning work practices. It was hoped that primary nurses would have a Diploma in Nursing or have undertaken the ENB 870 course.

For Smith Ward, it was important that new nurses were patient centred.

Ideal recruits would be 'practical allrounders', prepared to 'muck in' and not be status conscious. They were less likely to be interested in academic nursing and should not be overly idealistic, as they would only experience frustration in the face of the ward's working conditions. Often those candidates with a varied background rather than a straight nursing career path appeared more suitable. A sense of humour was of great importance. As with Jones Ward, intuition played an important part in staff selection. It was important that nurses should come across as 'a bit tender', with some indication that they had given thought to their beliefs or value system; a 'humanistic streak' was essential, whether or not the candidate had religious beliefs. At the same time, likely candidates would possess a degree of 'aggression' that enabled them to 'be themselves', to be 'blunt' in their dealings with people and 'to let off steam', rather than being robotic or likely to 'bottle things up'.

From this it appears that, to some extent, what the different wards looked for in new members of staff reflected local conditions within each hospital. But, in turn, the different qualities sought by each ward also helped to shape different operational styles for each nursing team. Jones Ward had what could be termed a 'visionary' approach, in which innovation was central in the pursuance of quality patient care and the development of nursing. In contrast, nurses on Smith Ward practised according to a 'pragmatic' approach, in which the availability of resources shaped their aspirations and activities.

It was clear, for example, that the existence of a distinct operational style helped to shape the choices made on each ward concerning organisational mode. Until impelled to implement the 'named nurse' initiative, Smith Ward retained patient allocation in the face of pressure to change, largely because of the constraints imposed by the ward's geography; the layout was such that there was greater potential for continuity of care with patient allocation than with team nursing, if male and female patients were to be nursed in separate bays. Thus, pragmatic considerations (the ward's layout) largely determined the mode of organisation.

This approach contrasted with that of Jones Ward, which, after the fieldwork period, was moved to new premises endowed with many of the features of Smith Ward. Most pertinently for this example, Jones Ward became a mixed-sex ward, composed of a number of bays and cubicles. In order to maintain continuity of care *and* the primary nursing mode of organisation, patients of both sexes were nursed side by side within each bay, although this was clearly unacceptable to some, who refused admission. Here nurses' vision of nursing was prioritised above pragmatic considerations.

The issues of ward style and local conditions, and the relationship between these, are of central importance to the findings of this study and will be discussed more fully in Chapter 10. This chapter has sought to show that nurses' choice of 'ward style' can be associated, to some extent, with their support needs. Nurses on Smith Ward developed a style of practice that helped them to cope with the lack of resources available to them, while, initially, nurses on Jones Ward were not hampered by this consideration. Yet towards the end the study, and since its completion, profound changes have taken place, which affected many aspects of the ward, including its resourcing. Significantly, once nurses on Jones Ward were no longer able to practise according to their 'visionary ethos', their support needs not only changed, but also went largely unmet. As a result, many permanent members of staff were thrown into professional and personal crisis.

10

Conclusion

Research does not take place in a vacuum, and this chapter will relate the findings of the study to ideological and political change that is taking place more generally. While the research this book describes was prompted by curiosity about the meanings of 'closeness' and concern regarding its implications for nurses, the impetus for the book itself was provided by the enormous changes currently occurring in the health service. Thus, this chapter will offer a summary of the research findings, a brief account of what has happened to the two wards since the end of the study and how we might view these changes, as they are clearly not unique to the hospitals in the study. Moreover, they suggest serious discrepancies between, on the one hand, the expectations of nurses and nursing, as made explicit, for example, in *The Patient's Charter* (Department of Health 1991) and, on the other, the extent to which such expectations can be met in the context of a market-led health service. Before this, however, we will consider the methodological approach underlying the study and clarify the way in which this is 'anthropological'.

NURSING AND ANTHROPOLOGY

As a nurse and an anthropologist, I have tried to use this book as an opportunity to show the relevance of anthropology for nurses and nursing. An increasing number of nurses are becoming interested not only in the social sciences generally, but also in what anthropology may have to offer them; however, there is, as yet, little anthropological material available to them that is specifically nursing-oriented. Anthropology is often characterised by cross-cultural comparison and, for many nurses, has become synonymous with transcultural nursing. This might be characterised, rather crudely, as the provision of culturally-sensitive care by reference to what are seen as the relevant features of different cultures.[1] Here I have tried to indicate other ways in which anthropology might be useful to nurses; what makes this study 'anthropological' is its focus and methodological approach.

In terms of focus, anthropology is highly diverse, but it is often concerned with how cultural groups understand their world through the study of the symbols they create. This research came to concentrate on the ambiguity of the nurse's world and how this ambiguity is managed. It deals, for instance, with how nurses manipulate the space they inhabit and the symbolic meanings they give to this space.

In terms of methodology, anthropology is characterised by an ethnographic approach and an emphasis on participant observation. There is, however, an increasing interest in refining participation, to concentrate on lived experience, so that, for example, knowledge derived from visual observation is not automatically given more weight than that which is sensed through the body. The self itself is viewed as participant, being changed by, as well as changing, the experience of others. Unlike in traditional empiricism, in which a boundary is drawn between the observer and the observed, in the 'radical empiricism' described by the anthropologist Michael Jackson (1989), the interaction between these parties becomes crucial. Yet radical empiricism stresses not only the ethnographer's interactions with those he or she studies, but also that knowledge is grounded in practical and participatory experience as much as observation. Thus, if bodily practices 'mediate a personal realisation of social values' (Jackson 1989, p.131), learning how others use the body may lead to a new understanding of their verbal statements and ethical views.

This research is informed by a 'radical empiricism' in order to study aspects of nurses' knowledge and practice that often pass unnoticed and are difficult to articulate. Accordingly, data collected through participation are given the same sort of weight that verbal data usually enjoy. This seems an important emphasis for a study that was always concerned with interaction between nurses and patients and which came to include nurses' lived experience of the body. It also seems an appropriate approach for the study of nursing more generally, as practitioners are increasingly aware of the significance of resisting a mind–body dualism in the development of theory and practice.

SUMMARY OF THE RESEARCH FINDINGS

In earlier chapters, it was explained that the study came to be concerned with how nurses understood the concept of 'closeness'. This notion of 'closeness' was important because it appeared to inform much of the 'new nursing', if not nursing more generally. The study also aimed to explore whether or not nurses received adequate support to sustain them in their 'close' relationships with patients, if and when these relationships developed.

In addressing these concerns, the study explored aspects of nurse–patient interaction, particularly through nurses' use of the body within a specific political and symbolic space. Nurses found the notion of 'closeness' difficult to explain, but it very often suggested to them a 'proximity' and a position from which it was possible to become 'open' or to 'open up'. Such 'openness' appeared to be central to the therapeutic element of nurse–patient interaction, with 'closeness' a precondition for this. In this sense, the way in which nurses used 'closeness' was reminiscent of Peplau's work, in which she suggests that 'closeness' is a matter of becoming 'closer to the truth of that person's current dilemma' (1969, p.352). From observation and informants' statements, however, it seemed that such 'proximity' should be understood in both physical and existential terms; an existential 'closeness' was expressed and fostered through physical proximity, and this, in turn, might itself be the grounds of a more metaphysical 'closeness' – as in the provision of intimate care. Thus, physical and non-physical dimensions of 'closeness' appeared to be mutually constituted and sustained, in a way that should perhaps not be surprising given the extent to which these dimensions are intertwined in nursing practice.

Just as family relationships are often based on a notion of 'closeness' (Savage 1991), those relationships nurses developed with patients that were characterised by 'closeness' often seemed to bear some resemblance to ideal family relationships. Particularly on Jones Ward, where nursing care was explicitly based on the 'closeness' between nurse and patient, nurses often described *good* nursing care as that which they offered *as if* the patient were a member of their own family.

This is suggesting something more than that nurses, in transforming patients into 'family', were simply professionalising women's domestic roles. Nurse–patient relations have been seen by some social scientists to resemble power relations between women and children in the patriarchal family; the good nurse has traditionally been equated with the good woman and the good mother (Gamarnikow 1978), but she has not been without power (Hugman 1991). Yet on Jones Ward (and, to some degree, on Smith Ward), nurses sought to create partnerships with patients in ways that inevitably undermined the power that nurses have traditionally held. Significantly, nurses on Jones Ward were often cast by patients as a daughter or sibling and not a mother.

'Familialisation' or domestication of the context of care was effected by nurses on Jones Ward through a number of means, including the reduction of ward routine, redrawing the boundary between nurses' and patients' space, the use of relaxed posture and changes in uniform style. Some of these measures, such as the development of a particular posture, were introduced without any apparently *conscious* intent to influence the nurse–patient relationship. They are, therefore, helpful in demonstrating elements of the embodied knowledge that nurses draw upon in the course of their work.

While nurses were clearly skilled in facilitating 'close' relationships through a range of practices, such relationships might vary in their emotional charge – in other words, they were not *necessarily* emotionally intense. It was unusual, for example, for nurses to see patients beyond the hospital setting, once the patient was discharged; relationships were defined and managed in the context of the hospital ward and would perhaps not have been sustainable in other settings. Thus, what was observed was not so much nurses' emotional labour (Smith 1992) but their labour to determine the *context* of nursing care, a context that would facilitate a therapeutic outcome for the patient without great personal cost for the nurse.

'Close' relationships might have involved different degrees of emotional involvement, yet it was apparent that nurses expressed no specific support needs as a result of the 'close' relationships they developed with patients. This does not mean that nurses did not need any support in this respect, but it seemed that any needs were largely being met and, therefore, remained implicit rather than explicit. It was clear, for example, that nurses found that the unspoken support they received from the rest of the ward's nursing team helped to sustain them in their practice.

Instead of finding that 'close' relationships left nurses in need of support, rather the reverse was found – that 'closeness' developed where nurses were well supported and did not develop to the same degree where support was weak. Nurses on Smith Ward found it stressful that they were unable to spend as much time with patients as they wished. Insufficient resources, such as shortages of nursing or ancillary staff, meant that nurses spent more time on non-nursing duties. On Jones Ward, nurses initially derived a high degree of satisfaction from their work. They were pleased to be able to spend a large proportion of their time on nursing duties. Their morale was lifted by the reciprocal nature of their relationships with patients, and the concern expressed by patients for nurses' welfare represented a significant source of support. What was stressful, however, were changes in the nature and resourcing of nurses' work that occurred during the study, which prevented nurses from sustaining the 'close' relationships they had established with patients.

EVENTS SINCE THE END OF THE STUDY

The two wards that were involved in the research no longer exist as described. Sweeping changes have occurred, which I have learnt about through conversations with members of the nursing staff, rather than through direct observation.

Smith Ward has been relocated to a different site and has become a single-sex ward with a Nightingale layout and 17 beds. Patient allocation has disappeared. There have also been other changes, concerning, for example, skill mix ratios and staffing levels. During the study, two posts for D grade nurses were frozen. Later, this number had increased to six. A greater proportion of agency nurses was being employed to counter the low staff levels, but as one of the senior nurses pointed out, having a large number of non-permanent staff changes the nature of the ward team. For instance, it becomes impossible to involve all staff in decision-making, and thus the way in which the ward is run becomes less democratic. At the same time, nurses' support needs may go unmet because knowing colleagues and being able to recognise when they are upset or stressed becomes more difficult.

Jones Ward went through a number of changes in location during the 18 months following the study. First a single-sex ward with a Nightingale lay-out, it became a mixed-sex ward comprising a number of four- and six-bedded bays, and then a mixed-sex Nightingale ward, before its current manifestation as an open-plan, usually single-sex ward. Whereas before there was a 'flattened hierarchy' (see Chapter 4, Figure 6), prompted by the wish for nurses to retain some clinical role as they became more senior, there is now a more traditional hierarchy, with a ward sister in overall charge. The original staff, many of whom had worked together for some years, have now left, mostly as a result of stress or dissatisfaction. These leavers include all the primary nurses. Ultimately, changes in nursing administration personnel, inadequate staffing levels, increased non-nursing duties and/or quasi-medical tasks (such as the administration of intra-venous antibiotics) and lack of support from senior staff and medical col-leagues contributed to many staff on Jones Ward feeling that they were unable to provide the kind of care they wished to give.

Care is now delivered through the organisational mode of team nursing. The ward has a large central nurses' station where nurses congregate to write notes; handovers mostly take place in a separate office, and nurses' use of relaxed body posture is less marked. The 'domestic space' has been largely institutionalised. It is impossible to say what has happened in terms of how nurses see their interactions with patients and the extent to which these are based on 'closeness', nor can any comment be made on how nurses perceive their nursing style and whether, for example, they still aspire to practise the 'new nursing'.

LOCAL INITIATIVES AND GOVERNMENT RHETORIC

The complexity of nursing is often not obvious to the outside observer. Although 'good nursing care is often demonstrated by the fact that you can't see it' (Royal College of Nursing 1992b) nursing's cost-effectiveness is often calculated on the basis of what is observable and measurable (Hart 1991, Hancock 1993). When nursing care becomes in any way visible, it is generally through seemingly simple tasks, such as bathing, which are the only tangible signs of a specific and often experiential form of knowledge (Benner and Wrubel 1989; Lawler 1991). Non-nurses generally assign little value to such tasks (see for example Dyson 1991), partly because their underlying meaning is not grasped and partly because such tasks may be seen as little more than an extension of women's domestic role (Attridge and Callahan 1989). Any recognition of nursing's value has been hampered by its history as an occupation for women, with, for example, nurses' skill in providing comfort interpreted as their *natural* helpfulness rather than the result of specific skills and knowledge (Strauss et al 1985). In other words, failure to recognise nurses' specific knowledge has to be understood in the context of the social construction of nursing as women's work.

There is no appropriate language to express the experiential, intuitive and creative dimensions of nursing (Hart 1991), but this is not the result of chance; there is a link between language use and sexual inequality:

> when people talk to each other they are engaged in an important political activity in which existing power relations dictate the way in which social reality is renegotiated among participants (Graddol and Swann 1989).

Thus, Hart found in a study of staff retention and turnover that nurses, who are often highly articulate among their peers, become reticent to speak in the face of other health service personnel. She notes (1991, pp.21–2):

> Anthropological literature contains many examples of the mutedness of one group in the face of another perceived to be more powerful. It is not that nurses do not speak: reticence comes about because what they have to say is not valued by those in power and is not listened to.

It is hoped that one contribution of the present study is to help to describe some of the elements of nursing that have gone largely unrecognised, and thus to increase the range of vocabulary available to nurses in their dealings with health service managers, purchasers and other powerful groups.

Additionally, in writing up the study, I set out to record something that has been lost. The book describes the endeavours of nurses on two wards to provide a patient-centred form of care and how these endeavours have been overturned, willingly or unwillingly, by those who have carried out recent health service policy. Jones Ward, in particular, has changed beyond recognition. At first glance, this may represent a fairly minor event in the face of swingeing health care 'reforms'; it has become commonplace to read of ward closures, nurse unemployment and reduced services for patients in the name of rationalisation. Yet putting these rather more quantifiable kinds of loss on one side, I shall concentrate on what the loss of Jones Ward means in terms of nursing's future overall.

Recent policy initiatives and strategies concerning the provision of health-care services have been seen by some to suggest that nursing is to take a central role in the future. For instance, the 'named nurse' initiative proposed within *The Patient's Charter* (Department of Health 1991) has been interpreted as a recognition of the value of nursing (Hancock 1992). Such proposals stress the importance of individualised patient care and, thus, of necessity, continuity of care. As the Audit Commission has said (1992, p.13):

> Continuity and patient-centred care are so fundamentally intertwined that it is difficult to say where one begins and the other ends. In order to see the benefits of detailed, individualised care planning, individual nurses need to have continuous relationships with individual patients.

Indeed, the Audit Commission states that they base their assessment of quality care on the degree to which care is continuous and individualised. Thus, although the Audit Commission does not go so far as to say that nurse–patient interaction may have therapeutic potential, it does suggest that the nurse–patient relationship is of huge importance in the provision of high-quality patient care.

This same Audit Commission report describes the ideal ward environment for bringing about improvements in patient care in the following terms (p.10):

> one of the signs that tells the visitor a great deal about the ward is its atmosphere. Where the individual patient is at the centre of nursing activity the atmosphere invariably appears to be calmer and less frenetic than on other wards. Nurses seem not to be rushing around looking so busy that it would have to be a brave patient indeed who asked for their attention. Nor do they sit in groups together, on the ward or in the office, recovering from the rush over cups of coffee and tea. Instead the pace of their work appears to proceed more steadily. No doubt they are busy, but they appear more in control and the pace of work is more even. It is also more common to see them sitting with patients without necessarily 'doing' anything to or for them, simply sitting and talking.

What is ironic about this description is that it fits Jones Ward as it existed during the study. Jones Ward had already introduced many of the measures proposed by the Audit Commission for ensuring continuous, patient-centred care (see Section 5 of the Audit Commission's report (1992)), long before the publication of the handbook. Despite innovative practice that prefigured government policy and addressed many of the objectives later annunciated by bodies such as the Department of Health (1989), the Audit Commission (1992) and the NHS Management Executive (1993), the staff of Jones Ward were prevented from continuing what has come to be regarded as good practice because of competing initiatives, primarily the introduction of an internal market. These other initiatives prompted changes, such as new skill mix ratios, designed to cut costs and make services offered by the hospital more attractive to purchasers of health care.

Unfortunately, there is nothing unique about the experience of nurses on Jones Ward. Increasingly, nurses everywhere are exhorted to develop 'good practice' but are caught between two opposing views of nursing. According to one view, reflected in *The Patient's Charter* (Department of Health 1991) or the reports of the Audit Commission, for example, the experience of health service consumers is paramount. By officially placing individualised care and continuity of care at the centre of nursing practice, a form of nursing based on the nature of the nurse–patient relationship is promoted – a form that is akin to the 'new nursing'.

The other view has its roots in the government initiative to transform the NHS into an internal market. In this view, perceptions of nursing are shaped by what is cost-effective. For example, nurses are seen as ideally placed to take on a range of what have previously been seen as medical tasks (such as routine intravenous injections). At the same time, they are pressurised into relinquishing traditional nursing care (such as bathing), which can be carried out more cheaply by untrained personnel. Here nursing is task oriented rather than patient oriented. Caught between these two views of nursing, many nurses find they are required to offer patient-oriented care on the basis of resources determined by a task-oriented approach.

In this context, there must be serious doubts as to whether basing nursing care on 'closeness' is a sustainable nursing option. This is not, after all, because of the emotional costs that nurses might have to bear but because the resources are not always available to sustain such patient-focused care. In the present political and economic climate, widespread adoption of the principles of the 'new nursing', such as a 'close' nurse–patient relationship, may just not be viable, despite the rhetoric of policy initiatives.

ENDNOTES

1. Critics of transcultural nursing have suggested that it represents little more than a 'menu' approach, in which the needs of the individual are largely determined by the characteristics attributed to the cultural group to which they are ascribed (Bruni 1988, Mason 1990). Because of this, transcultural nursing has been charged with ignoring the dynamic and heterogeneous nature of cultures, and with *perpetuating* cultural stereotypes and the ethnocentrism of nurses providing care.

Appendix

Key Characteristics of an NDU

A Nursing Development Unit can be established in any nursing, midwifery or health visiting setting in either the public or private sector. Whatever the area of practice, the NDU must fulfil the following criteria:

- be a defined clinical area where care is given directly to patients/ clients, or be an identified nursing team;

- have a clearly defined clinical nursing leader who has day to day responsibility and authority for clinical practice in the unit. This leader has a democratic management style and acts as the major change agent in the unit;

- have a philosophy of care which is developed collectively and is underpinned by a shared vision of high quality nursing practice and espouses the values of equity and equality in care;

- use an approach that increases the involvement of patients/clients in decision making regarding their own care;

- be a place where staff accept change as a way of life and take a proactive, dynamic, challenging and planned approach to management of change. NDU nurses experiment constantly to improve practice and develop themselves;

- require all nursing staff within the unit to be involved with, and have ownership of, the on-going development of clinical practice. This depends on a high level of individual practitioner autonomy;

- adopt strategies and development programmes aimed at empowering individual nurses. These concentrate on developing personal growth, awareness and assertiveness and encouraging autonomy;

- place a strong emphasis on staff professional development regardless of grade or qualification. An NDU, therefore, has a good track

record of devoting designated time and human/financial resources
to this;

• have already established, or be in the process of planning, reliable
methods of evaluating the efficiency and effectiveness of nursing
care, particularly in terms of patient/client health outcomes, and
overall quality of service;

• share knowledge of new ways of practice at both a local and
national level and provide a demonstration site for other nurses
through exchange visits, seminars, workshops etc;

• encourage unit staff to develop research-based practice. This may
be their own research, anything from small projects to a formal
research programme, or may be the application and evaluation of
research done elsewhere.

(reproduced by kind permission of the Nursing Developments
Programme at the King's Fund Centre)

These guidelines were in use at the time of the research although they have
subsequently been revised by the King's Fund Nursing Developments
Programme.

References

Aamodt A (1991) Ethnography and epistemology: Generating nursing knowledge. In Morse J (ed.), *Qualitative Nursing Research: A Contemporary Dialogue*. Newbury Park, California: Sage.

Adair L (1992) Touch and the nurse. *Journal of Clinical Nursing*, **1**(1): 5–6.

Altschul A (1972) *Nurse–Patient Interaction: A Study of Interaction Patterns in Acute Psychiatry Wards*. Edinburgh: Churchill Livingstone.

Ardener S (1993) Ground rules and social maps for women: an introduction. In *Women and Space: Ground Rules and Social Maps*. Oxford: Berg.

Armstrong D (1983) The fabrication of the nurse–patient relationship. *Social Science & Medicine*, **14B**: 3–13.

Attridge C and Callahan M (1989) Women in women's work: Nurses, stress and power. *Recent Advances in Nursing*, **25**: 41–69.

Audit Commission (1991) *The Virtue of Patients: Making Best Use of Ward Nursing Resources*. London: HMSO.

Audit Commission (1992) *Making Time for Patients: A Handbook for Ward Sisters*. London: HMSO.

Barrett M and McIntosh M (1982) *The Anti-Social Family*. London: Verso.

Bartky S (1988) Foucault, femininity and the modernisation of patriarchal power. In Diamond I and Quinby L (eds.), *Feminism and Foucault: Reflections on Resistance*. Boston: Northwestern University Press.

Bartle J (1991) Caring in relation to Orem's theory. *Nursing Standard*, **5**(37): 33–6.

Bell C (1992) *Ritual Theory, Ritual Practice*. Oxford: Oxford University Press.

Benner P (1984) *From Novice to Expert: Excellence and Power in Clinical Nursing Practice*. Menlo Park, California: Addison-Wesley.

Benner P and Wrubel J (1989) *The Primacy of Caring: Stress and Coping in Health and Illness*. Menlo Park, California: Addison-Wesley.

Berg D and Smith K (1988) *The Self and Social Enquiry: Researching Methods*. Newbury Park, California: Sage.

Berger P and Luckman T (1967) *The Social Construction of Reality*. London: Allen Lane.

Binnie A (1987) Primary nursing – structural changes. *Nursing Times*, **83**(39): 36–7.

Bloch M (1991) Language, anthropology and cognitive science. *Man* (NS), **26**(2): 183–98.

Booth J and Davies C (1991) The management of change on a nursing development unit. *Nursing Practice*, **4**(2): 12–15.

Bowers L (1989) The significance of primary nursing. *Journal of Advanced Nursing*, **14**: 13–19.

Boyle J (1991) Field research: A collaborative model for practice and research. In Morse J (ed.), *Qualitative Nursing Research: A Contemporary Dialogue.* Newbury Park, California: Sage.

Bruni N (1988) A critical analysis of transcultural theory. *Australian Journal of Advanced Nursing*, **5**(3): 26–32.

Brykczyńska G (1992) Caring – a dying art? In Jolley M and Brykczyńska G (eds.), *Nursing Care: The Challenge to Change.* London: Edward Arnold.

Burton G (1979) *Interpersonal Relations: A Guide for Nurses.* London: Tavistock.

Campbell A (1984) *Moderated Love: A Theology of Professional Care.* London: SPCK.

Cannell F (1990) Concepts of parenthood, the Warnock Report, the Gillick debate and modern myths. *American Ethnologist*, **17**: 667–86.

Carper B (1978) Fundamental patterns of knowledge in nursing. *Advances in Nursing Science*, **1**(1): 13–23.

Chapman G (1983) Ritual and rational action in hospitals. *Journal of Advanced Nursing*, **8**: 13–20.

Chipman Y (1991) Caring: Its meaning and place in the practice of nursing. *Journal of Nursing Education*, **3**(4): 171–5.

Clark J (1991) Nursing as an intellectual activity. *British Medical Journal*, **303**: 376–7.

Code L (1988) Experience, knowledge and responsibility. In Griffiths M and Whitford M (eds.), *Feminist Perspectives in Philosophy.* Basingstoke: Macmillan.

Coser R (1959) Some social functions of laughter. *Human Relations*, **12**(2): 171–82.

Coser R (1960) Laughter among colleagues: A study of the functions of humour among the staff of a mental hospital. *Psychiatry*, **23**: 81–95.

Creyghton M (1982) The open body: notes on Khroumirian body symbolism. In de Josselin de Jong P and Schwimmer E (eds.), *Symbolic Anthropology in the Netherlands.* The Hague: Marinus Nijhoff.

de la Cuesta C (1983) The nursing process: From development to implementation. *Journal of Advanced Nursing*, **8**: 365–71.

Dahlberg A (1987) *Transcendence of Bodily Suffering: An Anthropological Study of English Catholics at Lourdes.* Unpublished PhD thesis, University of London.

Department of Health (1989) *Working for Patients.* London: HMSO.

Department of Health (1991) *The Patient's Charter.* London: HMSO.

Diers D and Leonard R (1966) Interaction analysis in nursing research. *Nursing Research*, **15**(3):225–8.

Douglas M (1966) *Purity and Danger: An Analysis of the Concepts of Pollution and Taboo.* London: Routledge & Kegan Paul.

Douglas M (1975) Jokes. In *Implicit Meanings: Essays in Anthropology.* London: Routledge & Kegan Paul.

Dunlop M (1986) Is a science of caring possible? *Journal of Advance Nursing*, **11**(6): 661–70.

Dwyer T (1991) Humour, power and change in organisations. *Human Relations*, **44**(1): 1–19.

Dyson R (1991) *Changing Labour Utilisation in NHS Trusts.* Keele: Department of Health/Centre for Health Management, Keele University.

Emerson J (1971) Behaviour in private places: sustaining definitions of reality in

gynaecological examinations. In Dreitzel H (ed.), *Recent Sociology*, 2. London: Macmillan.

Emerson J (1973) Negotiating the serious import of humour. In Birenbaum A and Sagarin E (eds.), *People in Places: The Sociology of the Familiar*. London: Thomas Nelson & Sons.

Ersser S (1991) A search for the therapeutic dimensions of nurse–patient interaction. In McMahon R and Pearson A (eds.), *Nursing as Therapy*. London: Chapman & Hall.

Ersser S and Tutton E (1991) *Primary Nursing in Perspective*. London: Scutari Press.

Estabrooks C and Morse J (1992) Towards a theory of touch: The touching process and acquiring a touching style. *Journal of Advanced Nursing*, **17**: 448–56.

Farrah S (1971) The nurse – the patient – and touch. In Duffey M, Anderson E, Bergersen B, Lohr M and Rose M (eds.), *Current Concepts in Clinical Nursing*, Vol. III. St Louis: Mosby.

Fernandez J (1986) *Persuasions and Performances: The Play of Tropes in Culture*. Bloomington: Indiana University Press.

Field D (1984) "We didn't want him to die on his own" – Nurses' accounts of nursing dying patients. *Journal of Advanced Nursing*, **9**: 59–70.

La Fontaine J (1985) Person and individual: Some anthropological reflections. In Carrithers M, Collins S and Lukes S (eds.), *The Category of the Person: Anthropology, History, Philosophy*. Cambridge: Cambridge University Press.

Fox S (1990) The ethnography of humour and the problem of social reality. *Sociology*, **24**(3): 431–46.

Gamarnikow E (1978) Sexual division of labour: The case of nursing. In Kuhn A and Wolpe A (eds.), *Feminism and Materialism: Women and Modes of Production*. London: Routledge & Kegan Paul.

Giovannetti P (1986) Evaluation of primary nursing. *Annual Review of Nursing Research*, **4**: 127–51.

Goffman E (1971) *The Presentation of Self in Everyday Life*. Harmondsworth: Penguin.

Graddol D and Swann J (1989) *Gender Voices*. Oxford: Blackwell.

Graham H (1983) Caring: A labour of love. In Finch J and Groves D (eds.), *A Labour of Love: Women, Work and Caring*. London: Routledge & Kegan Paul.

Hammersley M and Atkinson P (1983) *Ethnography: Principles in Practice*. London: Tavistock.

Hancock C (1992) Named nurse. Open letter to Royal College of Nursing members.

Hancock C (1993) Nurses work–cost effectively. *Nursing Standard*, **7**(26): 24–5.

Haraway D (1989) The biopolitics of postmodern bodies: determinations of self in auto-immune system discourse. *Differences*, **1**: 3–44.

Hart E (1991) Ghost in the machine. *Health Service Journal*, Dec 5: 20–2.

Hawkes T (1972) *Metaphor*. London: Methuen.

Hochschild A (1983) *The Managed Heart: The Commercialisation of Human Feeling*. Berkeley: University of California Press.

Hockey J (1990) *Experiences of Death: An Anthropological Account*. Edinburgh: Edinburgh University Press.

Hockey L (1976) *Women in Nursing*. Sevenoaks: Hodder & Stoughton.

Howe J and Sherzer J (1986) Friend hairyfish and friend rattlesnake: or keeping anthropologists in their place. *Man* (NS), **21**(4): 680–96.

Hugman R (1991) *Power in the Caring Professions.* Basingstoke: Macmillan.

Jackson M (1983) Knowledge of the body. *Man* (NS), **18**(2): 327–45.

Jackson M (1989) *Paths Toward a Clearing: Radical Empiricism and Ethnographic Enquiry.* Bloomington: Indiana University Press.

James N (1984) A postscript to nursing. In Bell C and Roberts H (eds.), *Social Researching: Politics, Problems, Practice.* London: Routledge & Kegan Paul.

James N (1989) Emotional labour: Skills and work in the social regulation of feeling. *The Sociological Review,* **37**: 15–42.

Johnson M (1989) The onset of human identity and its relationship to legislation concerning research on human embryos. *Ethical Problems in Reproductive Medicine,* **1**: 2–7.

Jourard S (1964) *The Transparent Self.* New York: van Nostrand Reinhold.

Kalisch B, Kalisch P and Scobey M (1983) *Images of the Nurse on Television.* New York: Springer.

Kirmayer L (1993) Healing and the invention of metaphor: The effectiveness of symbols revisited. *Culture, Medicine and Psychiatry,* **17**: 161–95.

Kitson A (1987) Raising standards of clinical practice – The fundamental issue of effective nursing practice. *Journal of Advanced Nursing,* **12**: 321–9.

Kleinman A (1992) Local worlds of suffering: An interpersonal focus for ethnographies of illness experience. *Qualitative Health Research,* **2**(2): 127–34.

Lakoff G and Johnson M (1980) *Metaphors We Live By.* Chicago: Chicago University Press.

Lawler J (1991) *Behind the Screens: Nursing, Somology and the Problem of the Body.* Melbourne: Churchill Livingstone.

Leininger M (1988) Leininger's theory of nursing: Cultural care diversity and universality. *Nursing Science Quarterly,* **1**(4): 175–81.

Littlewood J (1991) Care and ambiguity: towards a concept of nursing. In Holden P and Littlewood J (eds.), *Anthropology and Nursing.* London: Routledge & Kegan Paul.

Lorensen M (1983) Effects of touch on patients during a crisis situation in hospital. In Wilson-Barnett J (ed.), *Nursing Research: Ten Studies in Patient Care.* Chichester: John Wiley.

MacGuire J (1991) Tailoring research for advanced nursing practice. In McMahon R and Pearson A (eds.), *Nursing as Therapy.* London: Chapman & Hall.

Macleod Clark J (1983) Nurse–patient communication – an analysis of conversations from cancer wards. In Wilson-Barnett J (ed.), *Nursing Research: Ten Studies in Patient Care.* Chichester: John Wiley.

MacLoed M (1993) On knowing the patient: experiences of nurses undertaking care. In Radley A (ed.), *Worlds of Illness: Biographical and Cultural Perspectives on Health and Disease.* London: Routledge & Kegan Paul.

McMahon R (1991) Therapeutic nursing: Theories, issues and practice. In McMahon R and Pearson A (eds.), *Nursing as Therapy.* London: Chapman & Hall.

McMahon R and Pearson A (eds.) (1991) *Nursing as Therapy.* London: Chapman & Hall.

McMillan I (1993) A disturbing picture. *Nursing Times,* **89**(8): 30–4.

Manley K (1988) Evaluation of primary nursing in the ICU. *Nursing Times,* **84**: 57.

Manthey M (1992) *The Practice of Primary Nursing.* London: King's Fund Centre.

Marriott M (1976) Hindu transactions: Diversity without dualism. In Kapferer B (ed.), *Transaction and Meaning: Directions in the Anthropology of Exchange and Symbolic Behaviour.* Philadelphia: Institute for Study of Human Issues.

Mason C (1990) Women as mothers in Northern Ireland and Jamaica: A critique of the transcultural nursing movement. *International Journal of Nursing Studies,* **27**(4): 367–74.

Mauss M (1973) Techniques of the body. *Economy and Society,* **2**: 70–88.

May C (1990) Research on nurse–patient relationships: Problems of theory, problems of practice. *Journal of Advanced Nursing,* **15**: 307–15

May C (1991) Affective neutrality and involvement in nurse–patient relationships: Perceptions of appropriate behaviour among nurses in acute medical and surgical wards. *Journal of Advanced Nursing,* **16**: 552–8.

May C (1992) Individual care? Power and subjectivity in therapeutic relationships. *Sociology,* **26**(4): 589–602.

Mead D (1991) Research report: Defining primary nursing as a basis for comparison. *Nursing Times,* **87**(17): 71.

Meerabeau L (1992) Tacit nursing knowledge: An untapped resource or a methodological headache? *Journal of Advanced Nursing,* **17**: 108–12.

Melia K (1981) *Learning and Working: The Occupational Socialisation of Nurses.* London: Tavistock.

Menzies I (1970) *The Functioning of Social Systems as a Defence Against Anxiety* (Reprint of Tavistock Pamphlet 3). London: Tavistock Institute.

Meutzel P-A (1988) Therapeutic nursing. In Pearson A (ed.), *Primary Nursing: Nursing in the Burford and Oxford Nursing Development Units.* London: Chapman & Hall.

Moore H (1988) *Feminism and Anthropology.* Oxford: Basil Blackwell.

Morse J (1983) An ethnoscientific analysis of comfort: A preliminary investigation. *Nursing Papers: The Canadian Journal of Nursing Research,* **15**(1): 6–19.

Morse J (1991) Negotiating commitment and involvement in the nurse–patient relationship. *Journal of Advanced Nursing,* **16**: 455–68.

Mulaik J, Megenity J, Cannon R, Chance K, Cannella K, Garland L and Gilead M (1991) Patients' perceptions of nurses' use of touch. *Western Journal of Nursing Research,* **13**(3): 306–23.

Mulkay M (1988) *On Humour: Its Nature and Place in Modern Society.* Cambridge: Polity Press.

NHS Management Executive (1993) *A Vision for the Future.* London: HMSO.

Okely J (1992) Participatory experience and embodied knowledge. In Okely J and Callaway H (eds.), *Anthropology and Autobiography.* London: Routledge & Kegan Paul.

Ortony A (1979) Metaphor: A multidimensional problem. *Metaphor and Thought.* Cambridge: Cambridge University Press.

Overing J (1985) Today I shall call him "Mummy": Multiple worlds and classificatory confusion. In *Reason and Morality.* London: Tavistock.

Pearson A (ed.) (1988) Primary nursing. In *Primary Nursing: Nursing in the Burford and Oxford Nursing Development Units.* London: Chapman & Hall.

Peplau H (1969) Professional closeness. *Nursing Forum,* **8**(4): 342–60.

Phaneuf M (1976) *The Nursing Audit.* Norwalk: Appleton-Century-Crofts.

Qureshi H (1990) Boundaries between formal and informal care-giving work. In Ungerson C (ed.), *Gender and Caring: Work and Welfare in Britain and Scandinavia*. London: Harvester Wheatsheaf.

Radcliffe-Brown A (1940) On joking relationships. *Africa*, **13**: 195–210.

Ramos M (1992) The nurse–patient relationship. *Journal of Advanced Nursing*, **17**: 496–506.

Raudonis B (1992) Ethical considerations in qualitative research with hospice patients. *Qualitative Health Research*, **2**(2): 238–49.

Reed J (1992) Individualised nursing care: Some implications. *Journal of Clinical Practice*, **1**: 7–12.

Roberston M and Boyle J (1984) Ethnography: Contributions to nursing research. *Journal of Advanced Nursing*, **9**: 43–9.

Robinson J and Strong P (1990). *The NHS – Under New Management*. Milton Keynes: Open University Press.

Robinson V (1977) *Humour and the Health Professions*. Thorofare, NJ: Charles B Slack Inc.

Royal College of Nursing (1992a) Approaches to nursing care. *Issues in Nursing and Health*, 13.

Royal College of Nursing (1992b) *The Value of Nursing*. London: Royal College of Nursing.

Ruxton J (1988) Humour intervention deserves our attention. *Holistic Nursing Practice*, **2**(3): 54–62.

Salvage J (1985) *The Politics of Nursing*. London: Heinemann.

Salvage J (1990) The theory and practice of the 'new nursing'. *Nursing Times*, Occasional paper, **86**(4): 42–5.

Sapsford R and Abbott P (1992) *Research Methods for Nurses and the Caring Professions*. Buckingham: Open University Press.

Savage J (1987) *Nurses, Gender and Sexuality*. London: Heinemann.

Savage J (1991) *'Flesh and Blood': Notions of Relatedness Among Some Urban English Women*. Unpublished PhD thesis, University of London.

Savage J (1992) Is nurses' embodied knowledge gender specific? Paper presented to Association of Nurses and Anthropologists study day, April 29, Centre for Study of Primary Care, Steels Lane, London E1.

Savage J (1993) The new nursing: A view from the margins. *St. Mary's Past & Present League Journal*, **30**: 25–32.

Schechner R (1990) Magnitudes of performance. In Schechner R and Appel W (eds.), *By Means of Performance: Intercultural Studies of Theatre and Ritual*. Cambridge: Cambridge University Press.

Sciama L (1993) The problem of privacy in Mediterranean anthropology. In Ardener S (ed.), *Women and Space: Ground Rules and Social Maps*. Oxford: Berg.

Searle J (1979) Metaphor. In Ortony A (ed.), *Metaphor and Thought*. Cambridge: Cambridge University Press.

Simon J (1988) Humour and the older adult: Implications for nursing. *Journal of Advanced Nursing*, **13**: 441–6.

Smith P (1992) *The Emotional Labour of Nursing: How Nurses Care*. Basingstoke: Macmillan.

Spain D (1992) *Gendered Spaces*. Chapel Hill & London: University of Carolina Press.

Stoller P (1989) *The Taste of Ethnographic Things: The Senses in Anthropology.* Philadelphia: University of Pennsylvania Press.

Strauss A, Fagerhaught S, Syszek B and Weiner C (1985) *The Social Organisation of Medical Work.* New York: University of Chicago Press.

Street A (1992) *Inside Nursing: A Critical Ethnography of Clinical Nursing Practice.* Albany: State University of New York Press.

Sumners A (1990) Professional nurses' attitudes towards humour. *Journal of Advanced Nursing*, **15**: 196–200.

Swales J (1994) Quis Custodiet? *The Lancet*, Jan 29, **343**: 247.

Swanson K (1991) Empirical development of a middle range theory of caring. *Nursing Research*, **40**(3): 161–6.

Thomas C (1993) De-constructing concepts of care. *Sociology*, **27**(4): 649–69.

Thomas K (1991) Introduction. In Bremmer J and Roodenburg H (eds.), *The Cultural History of Gesture.* Cambridge: Cambridge University Press.

Thomas L and Bond S (1990) Towards defining the organisation of nursing care in hospital wards: An empirical study. *Journal of Advanced Nursing*, **15**: 1106–12.

Travelbee J (1971) *Interpersonal Aspects of Nursing*, 2nd edn. Philadelphia: FA Davies.

Ungerson C (1983) Why do women care? In Finch J and Groves D (eds.), *A Labour of Love: Women, Work and Caring.* London: Routledge & Kegan Paul.

Ungerson C (ed.) (1990) *Gender and Caring: Work and Welfare in Britain and Scandinavia.* London: Harvester Wheatsheaf.

Vaughan B (1992) The nature of nursing knowledge. In Robinson K and Vaughan B (eds.), *Knowledge for Nursing Practice.* Oxford: Butterworth-Heinemann.

Weiss M (1993) Besides manners: Paradoxes of behaviour in grand rounds. *Culture, Medicine and Psychiatry*, **17**: 235–53.

Weiss S (1988) Touch. In Fitzpatrick J, Taunton R and Benoliel J (eds.), *Annual Review of Nursing Research.* New York: Springer.

Weiss S (1992) Measurement of the sensory qualities in tactile interaction. *Nursing Research*, **41**(2): 82–6.

Wex M (1979) *Let's Take Back Our Space: 'Female' and 'Male' Body Language as a Result of Patriarchal Structures.* Berlin: Frauenliteraturverlag Hermine Fees.

Wharton A and Pearson A (1988) Nursing and intimate physical care – The key to therapeutic nursing. In Pearson A (ed.), *Primary Nursing: Nursing in the Burford and Oxford Nursing Development Units.* London: Chapman & Hall.

Wright S (1990) *My Patient – My Nurse: The Practice of Primary Nursing.* London: Scutari Press.

Wright S (1991) Facilitating therapeutic nursing and independent practice. In McMahon R and Pearson A (eds.), *Nursing as Therapy.* London: Chapman & Hall.

Wright S (1992) The named nurse: A question of accountability. *Nursing Times*, **88**(11): 27–9.

Young C (1987) Intuition and nursing process. *Holistic Nursing Practice*, **1**(3): 52–62.

Young I (1990) Throwing like a girl: A phenomenology of feminine body comportment, motility and spatiality. In *Throwing Like a Girl and Other Essays in Feminist Philosophy and Social Theory.* Bloomington: Indiana University Press.

Index

Page numbers in **bold type** refer to figures; those in *italics* refer to tables. n after a page number indicates endnotes.

**Books are to be returned on or before
the last date below.**

LIBREX —